D1134664

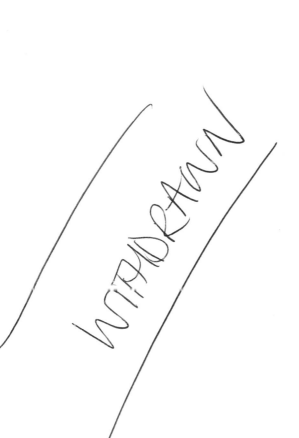

Understanding Physiotherapy Research

Understanding Physiotherapy Research

By

Chris Littlewood and Stephen May

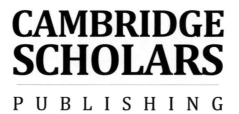

Understanding Physiotherapy Research,
by Chris Littlewood and Stephen May

This book first published 2013

Cambridge Scholars Publishing

12 Back Chapman Street, Newcastle upon Tyne, NE6 2XX, UK

British Library Cataloguing in Publication Data
A catalogue record for this book is available from the British Library

Copyright © 2013 by Chris Littlewood and Stephen May

All rights for this book reserved. No part of this book may be reproduced, stored in a retrieval system,
or transmitted, in any form or by any means, electronic, mechanical, photocopying, recording or
otherwise, without the prior permission of the copyright owner.

ISBN (10): 1-4438-4602-3, ISBN (13): 978-1-4438-4602-8

TABLE OF CONTENTS

LIST OF FIGURES

LIST OF TABLES

PREFACE

Why is there a need for another book about research? As experienced musculoskeletal physiotherapists involved in education and research we were aware of the difficulties that pre- and post-registration physiotherapists had in engaging with research evidence. In our experience, research is commonly treated as an add-on to physiotherapy educational curricula or clinical practice. The implications of research evidence are a concern only at the time of writing an assignment or preparing a presentation. It is something left largely to a minority with an interest. However, in an era of evidence based-practice, it is vital that all physiotherapists are aware of the inherent strengths and limitations of research studies and what this means for their practice. Despite this there is a dearth of physiotherapy specific texts that enable practising physiotherapists and students to effectively appraise and then apply research findings to their practice. Many generic research texts are available but, based upon our experience, this literature, which lacks a physiotherapy context, serves as a barrier to understanding and engaging with research.

To bridge this gap, this book presents a clinically focused range of methodological discussions in relation to specific research study designs in musculoskeletal physiotherapy. The intention of the book is to offer a platform upon which readers can develop their understanding of meaningful critical appraisal and hence gain confidence when reading published research. A focus on physiotherapy is preserved throughout the book to maintain engagement by discussing a topic of direct interest to the reader in a clinical language with which they are familiar. Our experience suggests that clinicians and students become lost when trying to apply abstract concepts from one topic to another. For those of you to which this sounds familiar, this book is for you. Our aim is to offer an introductory level text that is accessible and understandable to all those who appreciate the need to integrate research evidence into their practice, whether that is clinical, educational or managerial practice.

As with most substantial pieces of work, this book is not the product of the work of two individuals. We are indebted to our students, past and present, for asking the questions and subsequently stimulating the production of this book. We are also grateful to Ken Chance-Larsen, a friend and colleague, and Keith Hemsley, a friend and father-in-law, who took the time to review drafts of this work and offer helpful comments along the way.

CHAPTER ONE

EVIDENCE-BASED PHYSIOTHERAPY

Introduction

Everyone is now very familiar with the term evidence-based practice, a term that has been around for a number of years. Evidence-based medicine was a concept introduced in the 1990s and defined by one of its founders as "*the conscientious, explicit and judicious use of current best evidence*" (Sackett et al 1996). The background for this movement was that about only 15% of medical interventions were supported by solid scientific evidence, only 1% of articles were scientifically sound, and many treatments had never been assessed at all (Smith 1991). "*The weakness of the scientific evidence underlying (medical) practice is one of the causes of the wide variations that are well recognised in (medical) practice*" (Smith 1991). Subsequently the philosophy behind the concept was adopted by physiotherapists for very much the same reasons, and the term extended to become evidence-based practice / healthcare (Bury and Mead 1998).

It is important to make it clear from the start; evidence-based practice is not cook-book healthcare. Instead, evidence-based practice is about integrating the best available external evidence with clinical expertise and with patient preference (Sackett et al 1996). Thus external evidence is used but does not displace individual clinical expertise which should be used to determine if that evidence is relevant to the patient in front of you. It involves retrieving, appraising and, where appropriate, integrating that evidence to inform individual clinical decision making. As will become clear throughout this book, evidence does not just mean data obtained from randomised controlled trials and/or systematic reviews, though both are useful and important sources of evidence. The type of research evidence required will depend upon the clinical question being asked which in turn dictates the most appropriate form of research design required. If the question is about effectiveness of an intervention then, usually, a randomised controlled trial is the most appropriate research design; but if you want to find if a physical examination procedure is reliable between clinicians then a reliability study is necessary. If you want to find out about risk or prognostic factors for a certain disease then cohort studies are required. To find out about the perceptions held by patients or therapists then a qualitative study is needed. To find out if a physical examination procedure really does what the textbooks say it does, cross sectional studies comparing the test to a gold standard way of making that diagnosis would be appropriate. All of these study designs can be summarised and appraised in systematic reviews, so, for busy clinicians, these are an essential first read to get an overview on a topic.

Hierarchy of evidence

Sometimes the different study designs are ranked in a hierarchy of evidence, in which, for instance, systematic reviews are the strongest form of evidence, followed by randomised controlled trials, then cohort or case-control studies, then non-experimental studies, and lastly expert opinion (Gray 1997). Notice however that such hierarchies do not consider the type of question you are asking which, as stressed above, is central to the decision about the most appropriate study design to use. So, we suggest, it is best to take such hierarchies of evidence with a large pinch of salt, and *"you should never under any circumstances slavishly adopt or accept a hierarchy or grade of evidence"* (Earl-Slater 2002).

Implementing evidence-based physiotherapy

The founders of evidence-based healthcare described five procedural stages (Sackett et al 1997):

1) Formulate a clear clinical question based upon a patient's problem
2) Retrieve evidence with maximum efficiency to find evidence that addresses the question
3) Critically appraise that evidence for its validity (trustworthiness) and usefulness (applicability to your clinical setting)
4) Implement the findings into practice
5) Evaluate the impact of the evidence.

Obviously the research question will depend very much on the topic of interest that a patient has raised. Factors that might be relevant in your research question are: the type of patient you are interested in; the reliable and valid tools that are available in their assessment; reliable and valid outcome measurements; and effectiveness of interventions. From the research question you will develop key words, which should be directly relevant to the question, for instance, the type of patient group, the type of intervention, the outcomes of interest and the most applicable study design and so on. The acronym PICO (Higgins and Green 2008), sometimes supplemented with "S" to make PICOS, has been but forward as a useful reminder of these components and table 1.1 displays a basic search strategy structured around PICOS in response to the clinical question: *"Will mobilisation help my patient with low back pain return to work?"*

	Search terms
(P)atient group	Low back pain OR spinal pain OR lumbago
(I)ntervention	Mobilisation OR manipulation OR manual therapy
(C)omparator	Usual care OR physiotherapy OR placebo
(O)utcome	Return-to-work OR quality of life OR function
(S)tudy design	Randomised controlled trial OR randomized controlled design OR clinical trial OR systematic review

Table 1.1 Simple search strategy structured using PICOS

As seen from table 1.1, some key words and possible alternatives have been combined into search terms. It is appropriate to include as many synonyms as possible for each area of the search, and then combine them using the Boolean operator OR. This means that the electronic search will retrieve any papers that include these key words. The next step is to combine all the synonym terms with other aspects using the Boolean operator AND. This means that the electronic search should only retrieve papers that include the key words relating to the patient group **and** the intervention of interest **and** the outcome of interest etc. This is a way of restricting the search so that only potentially relevant papers are retrieved. Table 1.2 shows how this looks in practice.

Note in this example we have not included the terms for the comparator. In our experience of searching the physiotherapy-related literature this often significantly diminishes the return of the search meaning that important studies might be missed. By omitting the comparator terms, the worst-case scenario is that you will retrieve extra papers. In most cases this sensitive approach is preferable to one where a highly specific search excludes potentially relevant papers.

(low back pain OR spinal pain OR lumbago)
AND
(mobilisation OR manipulation OR manual therapy)
AND
(Return-to-work OR quality of life OR function)
AND
(Randomised controlled trial OR randomized controlled design OR clinical trial OR systematic review)

Table 1.2 Implementation of a simple search strategy

In terms of identifying the key words to include in the search, your own knowledge and experience is a starting point. However, this should be supplemented by looking at the key words of published papers, reviewing the search strategies of relevant systematic reviews and also adopting the work of others who might have developed a search strategy specifically related to the question you are asking or at least an aspect of the question you are asking, for example the Cochrane highly sensitive search strategy for identifying randomised trials (Higgins and Green 2008).

Once search terms have been identified then the next step is to identify electronic databases in which to implement the search. Relevant databases include the Medical Literature Analysis and Retrieval System Online (MEDLINE), Cumulative Index to Nursing and Allied Health Literature (CINAHL) and Excerpta Medica Database (EMBASE). Other important sources of evidence include the Cochrane database, which has its own series of systematic reviews, a Database of Abstracts of Reviews of Effectiveness (DARE), and the Physiotherapy Evidence Base (PEDro) which is a very useful source for physiotherapy related research, but is exclusively related to intervention studies, and not a good source for other types of evidence. PEDro though does have the added advantage of critically appraising the studies on the site and giving them a score out of ten for their methodology. Often a study scoring six or more out of ten is deemed to be high quality. However, if we stop to think, you might recognise that there is a certain amount of arbitrariness about determining the quality of a study in terms of a score out of ten. Imagine two studies, both scoring six out of ten and therefore both regarded as being of similar high quality. Now, for simplicity, what if one study meets criteria one to six and the second study meets criteria five to ten (what these criteria actually are is irrelevant at this stage)? The point to recognise is that the studies have both scored six out of ten but have met very different criteria to attain this. How can we be sure that meeting criteria one to six is the same in terms of study quality as meeting criteria five to ten? Currently we can't and this is why many have moved away from sole reliance on a quality score to determine the quality of a study.

Returning to the databases above; all are accessible online, although a subscription is required for some. We think it is useful to become familiar with the way they operate and their scope before commencing the search. A literature search of electronic databases, as described above, is frequently seen as a starting point by many and additional strategies, including contact with experts, searching the reference lists of the papers retrieved, hand-searching relevant journals and also citation-searching are useful complementary strategies to enhance the search.

Once the search has been implemented and the retrieved papers have been screened for relevance, the next stage is to undertake a critical appraisal. Critical appraisal refers to a process where you are asking: *"Can I trust the findings of these papers and if so are they applicable to my practice?"*

To facilitate the process of critical appraisal there are numerous published quality criteria available for all study designs (the PEDro tool for randomised controlled trials has been mentioned above). Currently it is unclear whether one quality appraisal tool or set of criteria is superior in a given situation. Despite this, there are some generally accepted quality issues that should be considered and these will be reviewed in subsequent chapters where relevant study designs are covered.

The next stage is implementation; straightforward in theory but potentially difficult in practice. Remember, evidence-based practice refers to integration of the best available external evidence with clinical expertise, and with patient preference. Consider a situation where a patient communicates a strong preference for ultrasound for the treatment of non-specific low back pain; *"it worked last time."* The research evidence points to exercise and restoration of function and cautions against the use of passive therapies, including ultrasound. You believe that ultrasound will do no harm but you also now believe that it will do no good. How do you proceed? The answer is not clear cut but attempts to prescribe an exercise programme to someone who does not believe in its potential, and hence is unlikely to engage with it, are unlikely to result in a favourable outcome. Clearly this is a challenge facing every clinician and one that has to be dealt with on an individual basis.

The final, or more accurately subsequent, stage of the evidence-based practice cycle is to evaluate impact. Remember, evidence-based practice is supposed to be superior to non-evidence-based practice. An on-going process of measurement is necessary to evaluate the impact of any changes.

Evidence-based physiotherapy in action

In this section we consider the use of therapeutic ultrasound and the evidence for its effectiveness. Therapeutic ultrasound is a modality taught at both undergraduate and postgraduate levels of physiotherapy and there is evidence from a number of studies from different countries that therapeutic ultrasound is considered a useful intervention. For instance, used by 8-22% of therapists in Britain, Ireland and Denmark for back pain (Foster et al 1999, Jackson 2001, Gracey et al 2002, Hamm et al 2003), 71% of therapists for back pain in Canada (Poitras et al 2005), 61% in Thailand (Pensri et al 2005), and about 5% in India (Fidvi and May 2010).

It has been claimed that therapeutic ultrasound has a number of properties, being both anti-inflammatory and an inflammatory stimulant at different intensities, and having the capacity to stimulate bone and soft-tissue healing (Norris 1997). The evidence for these properties comes largely from histological and tissue-based studies, rather than clinical practice. However, in the age of evidence-based practice, it is important to verify these claims in randomised controlled trials. Furthermore, unlike active physiotherapy interventions, such as exercise or manual therapy, blinding (the importance of this is discussed in subsequent chapters) of both patients and therapist is possible, and active ultrasound can be compared to placebo ultrasound. Thus the claims for its benefits should be scientifically verifiable.

Literature has been published relating to the effectiveness of ultrasound and twelve reviews are listed in table 1.3. It can be seen that the majority of reviews concluded that ultrasound was ineffective at treating soft tissue injuries, and compared to placebo had no effect on pain, swelling or healing times. The theoretical benefit from laboratory experiments did not carry over into the real world in a convincing way.

Remember, as stated at the outset of this chapter, the call for evidence-based practice arose from the weakness of scientific evidence for contemporary practice. So, in an era of evidence-based practice, why is therapeutic ultrasound still used when the weight of evidence provided over several decades demonstrates a lack of treatment effect compared to placebo? There are many possible reasons for this including patient and clinical preferences serving as barriers to implementation. However, a lack of confidence and technical ability in relation to critical appraisal are others. Thinking in relation to physiotherapy practice continues to evolve and it is no longer appropriate to rely on what we were taught. It is important that physiotherapists are aware of the inherent strengths and limitations of research studies and what this means for their practice. It is here where the focus of this book lies. Subsequent chapters revolve around critical appraisal of physiotherapy related research with the intention of offering a platform upon which readers can develop their understanding of meaningful critical appraisal, and hence gain confidence when reading published research and implementing research evidence into practice.

Conclusion

In this introductory chapter the aim has been to introduce or remind readers about some of the concepts behind research and evidence-based healthcare, and some of the motives for its introduction. We have examined an example of physiotherapy practice, therapeutic ultrasound, which has been retained in practice despite a lack of credible scientific evidence. As a profession it is important that our practice is truly evidence-based. The following chapters will review research evidence and different study designs with the aim of enhancing understanding and developing critical thought.

References

Alexander L, Gilman D, Brown D, Brown J, Houghton P (2010). Exposure to low amounts of ultrasound energy does not improve soft tissue pathology: a systematic review. Physical Therapy, 90, 14-25.

Baker K, Robertson V, Duck F (2001). A review of therapeutic ultrasound: biophysical effects. Physical Therapy, 81, 1351-1358.

Brosseau L, Casimiro L, Robinson V, Milne S, Shea B, Judd M, Wells G, Tugwell P (2001). Therapeutic ultrasound for treating patellofemoral pain syndrome. Cochrane Database of Systematic Reviews, Issue 4.

Bury T and Mead J (1998). Evidence-based Healthcare. Butterworth Heinemann, Oxford.

Chinn N, Clough A, Clough P (2010). Does therapeutic ultrasound have a clinical evidence base for treating soft tissue injuries? International Musculoskeletal Medicine, 32, 178-181.

Cullum N, Nelson E, Flemming K, Sheldon T (2001). Systematic reviews of wound care management: (5) beds; (6) compression; (7) laser therapy, therapeutic ultrasound, electrotherapy and electromagnetic therapy. Health Technology Assessment, 5, 9.

Earl-Slater A (2002). The Handbook of Clinical Trials and Other Research. Radcliffe Medical Press, Oxford.

Fidvi N and May S (2010). Physiotherapy management of low back pain in India – a survey of self-reported practice. Physiotherapy Research International, 15(3), 150-159.

Foster N, Thompson K, Baxter G, Allen J (1999). Management of nonspecific low back pain by physiotherapists in Britain and Ireland. Spine, 24, 1332-1342.

Gam A and Johannsen F (1995). Ultrasound therapy in musculoskeletal disorders: a meta-analysis. Pain, 63, 85-91.

Gracey J, McDonough S, Baxter G (2002). Physiotherapy management of low back pain. A survey of current practice in Northern Ireland. Spine, 27, 406-411.

Gray J (1997). Evidence-based Healthcare. How to Make Health Policy and Management Decisions. Churchill Livingstone, New York.

Hamm L, Mikkelsen B, Kuhr J, Stovring H, Munck A, Kragstrup J (2003). Danish physiotherapists' management of low back pain. Advances in Physiotherapy, 5, 109-113.

Higgins J and Green S (2008). Cochrane Handbook for systematic reviews of interventions. Wiley-Blackwell, Chichester.

Holmes M and Rudland J (1991). Clinical trials of ultrasound treatment in soft tissue injury: a review and critique. Physiotherapy Theory and Practice, 7, 163-175.

Jackson D (2001). How is low back pain managed? Physiotherapy, 87, 573-581.

Norris C (1997). Sports Injuries. Diagnosis and Management for Physiotherapists. Butterworth-Heinemann, Oxford.

Nussbaum E (1997). Ultrasound: to heat or not to heat – that is the question. Physical Therapy Reviews, 2, 59-72.

Pensri P, Foster N, Srisuk S, Baxter G, McDonough S (2005). Physiotherapy management of low back pain in Thailand: a study of practice. Physiotherapy Research International, 10, 201-212.

Poitras S, Blais R, Swaine B, Rossignol M (2005). Management of work-relates back pain: a population-based survey of physical therapists. Physical Therapy, 85, 1168-1181.

Robertson V and Baker K (2001). A review of therapeutic ultrasound: effectiveness studies. Physical Therapy, 81, 1339-1350.

Sackett D, Rosenberg W, Gray J, Haynes R, Richardson W (1996). Evidence based medicine: what it is and what it isn't. British Medical Journal, 312, 71-72.

Sackett D, Richardson W, Rosenberg W, Haynes R (1997). Evidence-based Medicine. How to Practice and Teach EBM. Churchill Livingstone, New York.

Smith R (1991). Where is the wisdom...? The poverty of medical evidence. British Medical Journal, 303, 798-799.

Van der Windt D, van der Heijden G, van den Berg S, ter Riet G, de Winter A, Bouter L (1999). Ultrasound therapy for musculoskeletal disorders: a systematic review. Pain, 81, 257-271.

Van der Windt D, van der Heijden G, van den Berg S, ter Riet G, de Winter A, Bouter L (2002). Therapeutic ultrasound for acute ankle sprains. Cochrane Database of Systematic Reviews, Issue 1.

Welch V, Brosseau L, Peterson J, Shea B, Tugwell P, Wells G (2001). Therapeutic ultrasound for osteoarthritis of the knee. Cochrane Database of Systematic Reviews, Issue 3.

Reference	Remit	N	Conclusions
Holmes and Rudland 1991	Soft tissue injury	18	Most studies were flawed, only one study with placebo found active US to be more effective.
Gam and Johannsen 1995	Musculoskeletal disorders	22	From meta-analysis of 13 studies no evidence that active compared to sham US gave pain relief.
Nussbaum 1997	Biophysical properties of US	Unclear	Evidence is contradictory and difficult to interpret. Efficacy of US still needs to be addressed.
Van der Windt et al 1999	Musculoskeletal disorders	38	11 / 13 placebo-controlled trials of good quality found no evidence that favoured US, except possibly lateral epicondylitis.
Baker et al 2001	Biophysical effects	Unclear	Not proven to have a clinical effect or do not occur in vivo.
Brousseau et al 2001	Patellofemoral pain	1	No clinical benefit.
Cullum et al 2001	Chronic wounds	10	Insufficient reliable evidence to draw conclusions.
Robertson and Baker 2001	Musculoskeletal disorders	35	8 / 10 studies of good quality active no better than placebo US; two suggested possible effect in CTS and calcific tendinitis.
Welch et al 2001	Osteoarthritis of the knee	3	1 / 3 was placebo controlled; none showed benefit.
Van der Windt et al 2002	Acute ankle sprains	5	4 / 5 placebo controlled trials showed minimal effect.
Alexander et al 2010	Soft tissue shoulder problems	8	Three studies showed significant benefit (two for calcific tendinitis); US at very high levels and long exposure.
Chinn et al 2010	Soft tissue injuries	7	2 / 7 placebo controlled trials showed benefit.

Table 1.3 Systematic reviews and reviews into the therapeutic effect of ultrasound (US); CTS = carpal tunnel syndrome

CHAPTER TWO

RESEARCH DESIGN

Introduction

Research design refers to the approach taken to answer a research question. In our experience deciding which research design to employ or deciding which research design has been used in a study presents a challenge to many. Most texts and critical-appraisal tools require that the reader has defined the research design before the relevant information can be accessed. For example, the Critical Appraisal Skills Programme (CASP) offers a range of critical-appraisal tools for a range of research designs; including the randomised controlled trial, cohort study, case-control study, qualitative study and others. However, this assumes that you are able to confidently recognise the research design before using or judging the quality of the study. Recognising the research design can be a challenge because a range of research designs are available to us but it is not always clear which designs should be used or have been used in published studies.

Different research designs have different roles and it is important that we recognise the relative merits of each. This might seem an obvious statement but the idea that the randomised controlled trial is the best research design to address all research problems is a common misconception that we encounter. Hence, this chapter will present some simple questions that any reader of research can ask to enable them to make a decision about the type of research design that should be or has been employed. Following this an overview of common research designs used within physiotherapy-related research will be presented as a means of introducing the forthcoming chapters. A schematic overview of these designs is presented in figure 2.1.

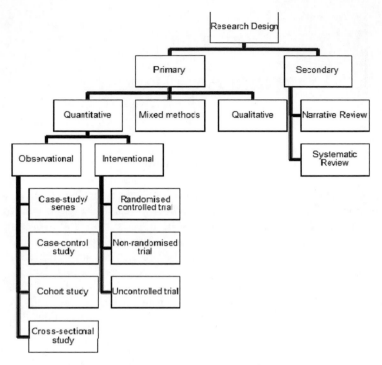

Figure 2.1 Overview of research designs

Primary or secondary research?

The first question to ask is whether the research is primary or secondary. Primary research studies collect data/ information directly from research participants. An example would be where researchers are interested to know how pain, associated with osteoarthritis of the knee, fluctuates over a one-year period. The researchers could recruit a group of people diagnosed with osteoarthritis of the knee and ask them to complete a questionnaire measuring the extent of pain at the beginning of the year and then after every three months. This is an example of a primary research question because data has been collected directly from the research participants.

Secondary research studies take a different approach to collecting data. These studies, often called reviews, collect data from primary studies. Secondary studies are most frequently undertaken to summarise the primary research that has been undertaken to date. This can be useful because it is important to understand what is already known before planning a primary study so that the study is capable of answering a useful research question and does not simply repeat what is already known. Also, because of the vast quantity of research that is produced, it is helpful to have a concise summary of research to enable clinicians to apply the evidence to their practice. So, a secondary research study could still aim to answer the same research question as a primary study but the approach to data collection is different. Hence the example of how pain associated with osteoarthritis of the knee fluctuates over a one year period could be a useful question upon which to base a secondary research study, but in this situation the study would identify primary studies that have investigated this area and summarise the findings from these studies.

Secondary research is further classified into either a narrative review or a systematic review (sometimes erroneously referred to as a meta-analysis). A narrative or non-systematic review is an approach where the author(s) selects primary studies, or possibly other reviews, to enable them to create their story. In contrast, the systematic review is expected to be conducted according to pre-specified methodological guidelines which the author(s) follows while constructing their review (Higgins and Green 2008). One of the key differences between these two types of reviews is that the author of a narrative review is not required to adhere to the same strict guidelines when selecting the studies they will use to inform their argument. Such freedom of selection leads many to question the validity or closeness to the truth of narrative reviews due to the high possibility of bias and it is mainly for this reason that fewer narrative reviews are now published.

Primary research; quantitative, qualitative or mixed methods?

If it is decided that the study to be evaluated or undertaken is primary research, then the next step is to consider whether it is qualitative, quantitative or mixed methodology.

Quantitative research

Quantitative data is straightforward to define and simply refers to the collection of numerical data; for example, age in years, weight in kilograms, exercise capacity in terms of maximum oxygen uptake, level of pain on a visual analogue scale. An example would be where researchers are interested to know whether physiotherapy reduces pain for people who complain of shoulder dysfunction. A measure of pain, for example the visual analogue scale, could be taken before treatment and then repeated after treatment to see whether a worthwhile change has occurred. In this situation a person may rate their pain as nine out of ten before treatment and four out of ten after treatment and so a numerical value equating to a five point change has occurred.

In the above example it is easy to see that numerical data is generated and so the study is regarded as quantitative. However, some studies might confuse as they blur the boundary between what is qualitative and quantitative data. Many quantitative studies use questionnaires to collect data. Some of these questionnaires, for example the Short-Form 36 (Ware and Sherbourne 1992), which is the most commonly used general health status questionnaire, ask research participants to mark a statement which most closely relates to their current situation. For example, a question asks: "*Compared to one year ago, how would you rate your health in general now?*"

The possible responses include;

- *much better than one year ago*
- *somewhat better than one year ago*
- *about the same, etc.*

Clearly this is not numerical but the responses are converted to numbers. So, the first response would equate to a score of one, the second response would equate to a score of two etc. Here the qualitative statements have been used to inform the research participant of the range of responses but these responses are then assigned a numeric value and treated quantitatively.

Qualitative research

Qualitative research has been defined by different people in different ways but essentially this approach refers to research where non-numerical data is collected. Most frequently this data comes in the form of observation of actions or the spoken word (Pope and Mays 2000). An example would be where researchers are interested to know physiotherapists' attitudes to hand washing on a general surgical ward. When the range of possible answers is unknown or unclear, the researchers could interview the physiotherapists to help understand the range of possible attitudes, for example; "*it's a good thing and I do it all the time*"; "*it's a good thing but I don't always have the time*"; "*it's unnecessary so I don't bother.*" The data collected here would be the spoken word of the physiotherapist. This could then be followed up by using observation where the researchers could see whether what the physiotherapists said was the same as what they did.

Qualitative research is useful to provide depth to our understanding. For example, a quantitative study might demonstrate that, over time, an increasing number of patients do not attend physiotherapy appointments, but it does not explain the reason or reasons why this might be happening. A qualitative study might recruit those patients who did not attend and interview them to ask why.

Mixed methods research

Over recent years the use of mixed methods research has become more common. Mixed methods research has been defined as the integration of qualitative and quantitative research methods within a single study (Creswell and Plano Clark 2011). The example of non-attendance could be an example of a mixed methods study where the quantitative research highlights the problem and the qualitative study investigates the reasons underpinning this problem. Another common use of mixed methods research is where quantitative research is used to evaluate the effectiveness of a new treatment or intervention and qualitative research is used to understand how the treatment was delivered in practice, whether barriers were faced and, if so, how these were overcome.

The next section will focus upon some common sub-classifications of quantitative research because this is where most confusion seems to arise.

Quantitative; observational or interventional?

So, you have identified that numerical data has been collected in the research you are studying or that collection of numerical data is appropriate to answer the research question you have formulated. At this stage the next question is to ask whether the study is or will be observational or interventional/ experimental. Observational research describes a situation where the research participants *are not* exposed to treatment or intervention as part of the research. Interventional/experimental research describes a situation where the research participants *are* exposed to treatment or intervention as part of the research (Dawson and Trapp 2001). An example of observational research would be where researchers are interested to know whether people who attend pulmonary rehabilitation classes experience further functional improvement following discharge from the class. At the point of discharge a measure of function could be taken, for example the six-minute walk test, and this could be repeated at time intervals for as long as is required. During this follow-up period when the six-minute walk test is repeated, further medical treatment or rehabilitation might be accessed and received by the patient but this is independent of the research and not delivered as part of the study. Although this is a common source of confusion, this study is still observational in nature.

An example of interventional/ experimental research would be where researchers are interested to know whether people who attend additional pulmonary rehabilitation classes beyond those conventionally prescribed experience further functional improvement. At the point of completion of the standard number of classes and prior to beginning the additional classes, a measure of function could be taken, for example the 6-minute walk test. The research participants would then attend the additional classes as part of the research before another 6-minute walk test is repeated to determine whether further progress has been made. The key aspect here is that the additional rehabilitation would not have been received if the research had not been undertaken and so the research participants are exposed to treatment as part of the research and not as a part of usual care.

Classification of observational studies

Case-study/ Case series

A case-study is a report or a description of some or all aspects of a patient encounter. Usually this report will describe an uncommon clinical presentation (Chance-Larsen and Littlewood 2010), a novel approach to diagnosis or a treatment that would not typically be administered (Littlewood and May 2007). The role of a case-study is to introduce or highlight the rare case or novel approach for the interest of the wider clinical or research community. For some, a case-study would not be regarded as research but we include it here because these studies are frequently published and have a useful role in introducing rare conditions or novel approaches and as a basis upon which to begin to plan future research.

A case-series is basically an extension of the case-study. The case-series consists of a report or a description of some or all aspects of a number of patient encounters. The role of the case-series is also similar to that of a case study but the meaning or implication arising from a case-series is greater due to the greater number of patients that are included.

Case-control study

The case-control study is designed to investigate factors that might contribute to or protect from the development of a disease or condition. This design is not to be confused with the case-study or case series; they are distinct research designs with very different roles. The case-control study recruits a group of cases, meaning people with a condition of interest or diagnosis, and a group of controls, meaning people similar to those with the condition or diagnosis but without the specific condition. For example, a group of people with osteoarthritis of the knee could be recruited as cases along with a group of people without osteoarthritis of the knee but similar to the cases in terms of age, gender and socioeconomic status. The history of the cases and controls would then be examined to determine similarities and differences in terms of potential risk factors, meaning factors that might contribute to the development of the condition (Dawson and Trapp 2001). Using the example of osteoarthritis of the knee, factors including family history of osteoarthritis, diet and previous levels of sporting activity might be investigated retrospectively (looking backwards) through clinical records, interviews or questionnaires. If one factor, for example a family history of osteoarthritis, is more commonly reported in the group of cases then a conclusion suggesting an association between this factor and the development of osteoarthritis of the knee could be drawn. If one factor, for example a history of a Mediterranean-based diet, is more commonly reported in the group of controls then a conclusion suggesting an association between this factor and protection against osteoarthritis of the knee could be drawn. At this stage a word of caution; association does not mean causation and a case-control study is not the design to establish causality. So, a Mediterranean-based diet might be associated with less osteoarthritis of the knee but this does not mean that if people adopt such a diet that they will not develop the condition. Other factors, for example obesity, might be the true source of the problem. The issue of establishing causation will be discussed more in relation to the randomised controlled trial.

Cohort study

The cohort study refers to a process of data collection from people with shared characteristics, for example the same diagnosis (Herbert et al 2005). So, for example, a cohort study might recruit a group of people who consult their general practitioner complaining of low back pain. This cohort would be followed to see, for example, how the associated pain and disability change over time and how long it takes to recover. Such a cohort study has the potential to offer useful information relating to the natural history of low back pain which enables an understanding of the course of the condition and prognosis.

Cross-sectional study

In contrast to the cohort study which is regarded as longitudinal because it collects data over time, the cross-sectional study describes collection of data at one point in time (Herbert et al 2005). Most commonly a cross-sectional study would be used to describe current approaches to treatment of a clinical condition or would be used to investigate how common a clinical condition is or would be used to evaluate the diagnostic accuracy of a test or procedure. For example, a researcher might be interested to know how physiotherapists currently treat a clinical condition in order to plan an experimental study comparing a new treatment to an existing treatment. A cross-sectional study might also be used to investigate whether practice has changed from one time point to another, maybe in relation to a policy change or in response to publication of new guidance.

Classification of interventional studies

Randomised controlled trial

The randomised controlled trial is regarded by many as the most appropriate research design to evaluate the effectiveness of an intervention (Littlewood 2011). There are three key components to a randomised controlled trial and the clue is in the name. Firstly, the research participants are allocated to two or more groups *randomly*, meaning by chance. Secondly, in its most basic form, research participants are allocated to the intervention or *control* group. Thirdly, the intervention group is compared to the control group in order to evaluate whether one group has performed better than the other and hence whether one treatment is more effective than another (Torgerson and Torgerson 2008). Figure 2.2 offers a schematic representation of the randomised controlled trial.

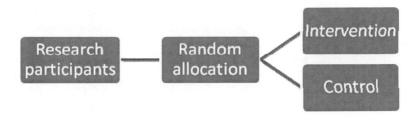

Figure 2.2 The randomised controlled trial

Taking the components of a randomised controlled trial in sequence, random allocation will be considered first. Imagine a physiotherapist who has designed a new exercise intervention for the treatment of low back pain and wants to establish the effectiveness of the treatment. She receives the first patient in the clinic; a young male with mild low back pain who continues to work and enjoys exercising. She decides that the patient should receive the new treatment and allocates him accordingly. The second patient of the day is also a young male but in contrast has not worked due to severe low back pain for a number of years and does not appreciate the benefits of exercise. She decides that this patient would probably not respond well to the new exercise intervention and so allocates him to the usual physiotherapy treatment. This non-random process of selection continues until all 100 research participants are recruited. Upon completion of the trial the physiotherapist notices that patients in the intervention group were more active and, on average, reported milder levels of low back pain. This means that the groups being compared are different to begin with, even before they are exposed to the treatment.

After the data is collected, the analysis suggests that the new exercise intervention is far superior to usual physiotherapy. Is this a valid conclusion? Probably not; because as physiotherapists we know that people with less severe pain, who maintain good levels of activity, tend to perform better than those with more severe pain and greater functional deficit, irrespective of the treatment they receive. This is an example of selection bias where the process of allocation of participants to groups has been adversely influenced. In contrast, a process of random allocation would serve to distribute participants between the group in a more balanced manner according to the factors we know, for example age, gender, condition severity; and the factors we don't know, for example psychological status, attitude to treatment. This provides a more appropriate basis upon which to judge the effectiveness of an intervention because the only significant difference between the groups should be the treatment received rather than other factors that can influence the outcome of treatment.

The second component, the control group, will now be considered. It is easiest to recognise the value of a control group by considering a situation where it is not used. Another example; following a day's lectures many students would complain of headaches. We would ask them to rate the severity of their headache on a scale of zero to ten where zero equates to no pain and ten equates to the worst pain imaginable. We would then instruct them regarding an exercise intervention that we spent many months developing; repeatedly elevating their left arm. We were not sure why this intervention worked but we had spent so much time thinking about it that it had to be worth something. We would ask the students to repeat the exercise two or three times before returning the next morning. Consistently, we found that the severity of the students' headaches had reduced significantly by the following morning. Should we conclude that our exercise intervention is effective based upon this data? Clearly not, it is much more likely that not having to listen to our voice, doing something more enjoyable, having a good rest and other factors were more likely to explain the reduction in headache severity. If we had randomly allocated students with headache to the intervention group, who undertook the exercise, or control group where students continued as usual without the exercise then a more valid evaluation would be possible. When the students returned the following morning we could establish the headache severity of both groups knowing that the only difference between the groups was that one received the intervention and the other didn't because the control group would also be exposed to all these other factors, for example rest, that might be responsible for a reduction in headache severity. In this situation it is highly unlikely that our exercise intervention would prove its worth and hence the value of a control group is highlighted.

An important point to recognise in relation to physiotherapy research is that the control group does not usually consist of no treatment. The reason for this is that it is generally accepted that it is unethical to withhold treatment of potential benefit from patients. So most randomised controlled trials involving physiotherapy compare the new intervention against a placebo, for example de-tuned ultrasound, or usual care, for example usual medical care. Hence the new intervention is expected to demonstrate that it is at least equivalent but usually superior to existing treatment before it would be considered for implementation into practice.

The third component, the trial, simply refers to the process by which an intervention is evaluated. In a randomised controlled trial this evaluation is in comparison to the control or usual treatment and in other designs this evaluation might take place comparing data from one time point to another.

Non-randomised trial/ Quasi-experimental study

The non-randomised trial or quasi-experimental study has the second and third components of the randomised controlled trial but is significantly different because research participants are not allocated to the intervention or control group randomly. Other means of allocation are used, including the time at which the clinic was visited or the physiotherapist seen. The main drawback with this design is selection bias as discussed in relation to the randomised controlled trial. Figure 2.3 offers a schematic representation of the quasi-experimental study.

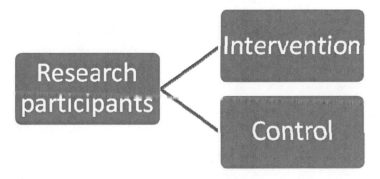

Figure 2.3 The non-randomised trial/ quasi-experimental study

Uncontrolled trial

The uncontrolled trial is also called a before-and-after study. Unlike the previous interventional studies described this study only has one group and hence lacks a process of random allocation and also lacks a control group against which the effectiveness of an intervention can be evaluated. Again, selection bias is a drawback here as is the lack of an appropriate control group against which a treatment can be adequately evaluated. Figure 2.4 offers a schematic representation of the uncontrolled trial.

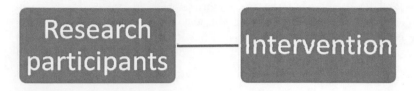

Figure 2.4 The uncontrolled trial

Summary

Although not exhaustive in terms of coverage, this chapter has introduced a range of commonly-used research designs. A process of deciding which design has or should be utilised has been described along with a brief introduction to the key features and uses of these designs. The following chapters will consider each of these designs in more detail, along with practical examples of each design taken from the published literature. These chapters will explore the features of each of these designs and explain the associated strengths and limitations before considering the implications for physiotherapy practice of the included studies.

References

Chance-Larsen K and Littlewood C (2010). A case of long thoracic nerve palsy. International Journal of Physical Therapy and Rehabilitation, 1, 41-43.

Critical appraisal skills programme (CASP). Available via: www.casp-uk.net.

Creswell J and Clark V (2011). Designing and Conducting mixed methods research (2nd edition). Sage publications; London.

Dawson B and Trapp R (2001). Basic and clinical biostatistics (3rd edition). McGraw-Hill; New York.

Herbert R, Jamtvedt G, Mead J, Hagen K (2005). Practical evidence-based physiotherapy. Elsevier' London.

Higgins J and Green S (2008). Cochrane Handbook for systematic reviews of interventions. Wiley-Blackwell, Chichester.

Littlewood C and May S (2007). A contractile dysfunction of the shoulder. Manual Therapy, 12, 80-83.

Littlewood C (2011). The RCT means nothing to me! Manual Therapy, 16, 614-617.

Pope C and Mays S (2000). Qualitative research in health care (2nd edition). BMJ publishing group, London.

Torgerson D and Torgerson C (2008). Designing randomised trials in health, education and the social sciences. Palgrave Macmillan, Basingstoke.

Ware J and Sherbourne C (1992). The MOS 36-item short-form health survey (SF-36): I. Conceptual framework and item selection. Medical Care, 30, 473-483.

CHAPTER THREE

QUALITATIVE RESEARCH

Introduction

The term qualitative research is somewhat of an umbrella term that, like quantitative research, describes a range of different approaches, such as ethnography and grounded theory. As mentioned in chapter two, qualitative research has been defined by different people in different ways reflecting the range of approaches associated with this paradigm. For the sake of clarity we will continue to use qualitative research as a singular term to refer to research where non-numerical data, for example observation of actions or the spoken word, is collected. We recognise that this simple approach does not reflect qualitative research in its entirety, but this is not the aim of this book. Instead we aim to offer a solid foundation upon which the novice researcher can develop their understanding.

Historically within physiotherapy, qualitative research has largely taken a back seat to the more dominant quantitative approaches (Petty et al 2012a). A variety of reasons have been proposed for this imbalance, including the argument that qualitative research lacks rigour and scientific credibility. Also, some have questioned the value of qualitative research due to difficulties generalising the findings from the research setting to clinical practice (Pope and Mays 2000). These concerns about qualitative research have been cited in the context of the physiotherapy profession aiming to establish its worth where the establishment of a worthwhile treatment effect is regarded as the holy grail, traditionally seen as the role of quantitative research.

However, as the limitations of quantitative research have become more apparent to health service researchers and the functions of qualitative research have become more appreciated, the quantitative/qualitative imbalance appears to be shifting (Petty et al 2012a). A recent example of our own work highlights this (Littlewood et al 2012a). We were interested in evaluating the effectiveness of a self-managed exercise programme versus usual physiotherapy for chronic rotator cuff disorders. For this purpose we selected a quantitative research design, a randomised controlled trial, where the treatment outcome from one group would be measured and compared against the other. This enables us to conclude that, on average, the intervention group (self-managed exercise) is superior, inferior or similar to the control group (usual physiotherapy). Hence, a possible conclusion might be that the treatment outcome of the self-managed exercise group was superior to usual physiotherapy; but this tells us nothing about the individual experience, an important concept for physiotherapists to understand. As with most interventions, as a research team, we expected different responses from different patients. Some might do better than they would if they had received usual physiotherapy, some might have a similar outcome, but for some the outcome might be worse. For research to be more useful to physiotherapists and their patients it would be helpful to explore possible reasons for the varied outcomes. Here qualitative research was used and individual patients and physiotherapists were interviewed to understand these reasons. If we had undertaken only quantitative research we would know which treatment was superior or otherwise, on average, but we would not know the reasons for this. For example, *"the exercise hurt so I didn't do it"* or *"I didn't have the time to do the exercise"* or *"I didn't have time to go to the clinic"* or *"I didn't understand what they were telling me"* or *"the exercise was great because I didn't have to go to the clinic, I could do it in my spare time and did not have to take time off work."* This rich qualitative data helps us to understand why an intervention might or might not work which then offers a basis upon which to develop it for use in clinical practice, if indicated by the outcome of the research, and for further evaluation in subsequent research studies.

Despite the clear benefits of mixing qualitative and quantitative methods, as shown in the above example, qualitative research does not always need to be used in this combined way. The research design should be informed by the research problem or question. Some research questions will require mono (one approach) rather than mixed methods research. With this in mind, qualitative research is used to describe or explore phenomena, including meaning and experience, in an in-depth way (Ritchie and Lewis 2003). To highlight this, the following section will offer a critical appraisal of three qualitative research studies that aimed to explore the meaning of patient satisfaction in relation to physiotherapy. All of the studies, summarised in table 3.1, explore a relatively complex area by attempting to determine the meaning of satisfaction from the patients' perspective.

Critical appraisal

The three studies to be appraised are: May (2001), Hills and Kitchen (2007) and Sheppard et al (2010). There is debate about the most appropriate way to judge the quality of a qualitative research study with some authors suggesting that it shouldn't be done, some authors suggesting it should be done using the same criteria as that used to judge quantitative research and some authors suggesting that it should be done but using criteria thought to be directly relevant to the qualitative paradigm (Spencer et al 2003). This account favours the latter approach and will discuss the strengths and weaknesses within this framework.

Research question/ aim

All three studies provided clear aims indicating their intention to explore patient satisfaction in different physiotherapy contexts. This is important to enable the reader to judge the relevance of the study and to also begin the process of quality appraisal. Where there is a clear statement of purpose the appropriateness of the research design, research methods and the data collected can be judged as a precursor to evaluating the overall *credibility, dependability, confirmability and transferability* of the research findings (Lincoln and Guba 1985). These terms are widely used in the language of critical appraisal of qualitative studies and will be explained in the forthcoming sections.

Research design

For the purpose of clarity, all three studies are regarded as being qualitative in nature. In this situation, a qualitative research design is appropriate for two main reasons which should be considered in tandem:

1) Due to the exploratory nature of the research,
2) Due to the complex nature of the phenomena under investigation.

Satisfaction is regarded as complex because it is likely to mean different things to different people and it is also likely to be multi-dimensional in nature. Patients are unlikely to be satisfied if they have to wait months to attend physiotherapy and then gain no benefit, even if they are treated by a warm, friendly and knowledgeable physiotherapist. Hence, in-depth exploration is needed to un-pick this complexity. Furthermore, before these studies were undertaken, similar research from a physiotherapy perspective was scarce and hence little was known about the range of factors that patients regarded as being important determinants of satisfaction. This means that it would be difficult and probably inappropriate to use other methods of data collection, for example a questionnaire which listed possible determinants of satisfaction and could be mailed out to patients to seek their opinion before counting up the responses and offering a numerical summary. This approach would not capture factors that are important to the patient and hence would not be regarded as *credible,* which refers to the accuracy of definition and description of the phenomenon under investigation. Clearly a qualitative approach is appropriate to offer in-depth exploration of satisfaction which contributes to the credibility of all three studies.

Sample/ context

All of the studies used purposive sampling to recruit participants. Purposive sampling is a non-random method of sampling which aims to identify people with a particular characteristic (Bowling 2002); in this case the characteristic was attendance at physiotherapy. Although commonly criticised for its non-random nature, purposive sampling is entirely appropriate for these qualitative studies. Consider the study by Sheppard et al (2010) where the concept of satisfaction in relation to the emergency department physiotherapist was investigated. If these researchers attempted to take a random sample of patients attending the emergency department then it is possible that their sample would be representative of all patients who attended the emergency department in that particular setting and hence any data they collected would be generalisable from their sample to the wider emergency department population. In principle this sounds good, but it is at odds with the aim of the research because some of those patients would not have experienced the physiotherapist during their time in the emergency department. It is more likely that they were managed by nursing and/or medical professionals. So, if these patients were interviewed they would have no comment to make about satisfaction in relation to the emergency department physiotherapist because they have no experience to draw upon. Random sampling in this context would be a waste of time because most patients would not have experience of the phenomena under investigation and so would not be able to discuss their experience. Qualitative research is concerned with depth of understanding and so information-rich participants are sought during the sampling process.

It will often be read that the aim of qualitative research is not to generalise the findings from the sample to the wider population. One philosophical reason for this is that one person's truth might not be the same as another's. For example, the factors that determine satisfaction for a wealthy middle-aged male living in rural England might be entirely different to those factors that determine satisfaction for a young homeless female. So, for many, generalisable findings are not valued in the qualitative paradigm. This philosophical argument could equally be applied to quantitative research.

However, a more immediate barrier to the generalisability of findings is the tendency for qualitative research to undertake non-random sampling, as described above, and recruit relatively low numbers of participants. These methodological decisions are entirely appropriate to enable recruitment of information rich participants and to undertake in-depth analysis of the data, but this means that the participants will not be sufficiently representative of the wider population. Hence, instead of qualitative research being judged in relation to whether the findings are generalisable it is more appropriate to consider whether the findings are *transferable*, which refers to the capacity to apply findings from one context to another (generalising would refer to applying the findings from one context to many contexts). Sheppard et al (2010) highlighted this issue. Their study refers to satisfaction with an emergency department physiotherapist within an inner city hospital in Australia. The role of this physiotherapist predominantly relates to care of the elderly, whereas in the UK this role predominantly deals with acute musculoskeletal injuries from all age groups. The context offered by Sheppard et al (2010) is a useful basis upon which a judgement regarding transferability can be made; *"is this context similar to mine?"* This thick description of the context facilitates such a decision and it becomes apparent that physiotherapists working in emergency departments in the UK might be cautious about transferring the findings from the study by Sheppard et al (2010) to their own practice settings.

Further to this, all three studies provided information relating to the setting of the research as well as demographic data, for example, age, gender, primary complaint, which enhances the *transferability* of the studies but ultimately individual readers need to make the decision in relation to their own practice.

Data collection

Thus far the approach taken by the three studies has been broadly similar but at this point divergence occurs. May (2001) collected data using individual interviews. Hills and Kitchen (2007) began with what they termed "developmental interviews" and then collected further data using focus groups. Sheppard et al (2010) employed a two stage process involving initial face-to-face interviews followed by telephone interviews.

May (2001) undertook semi-structured interviews, a common method used in qualitative research. Here the interviewer follows a set of pre-specified questions but allows the interviewee sufficient flexibility to tell their story within this framework. Individual interviews are useful when in-depth exploration of the experience of individuals is required (Petty et al 2012b). In this situation the use of individual interviews is appropriate and adds to the *credibility* of the study. However, a potential threat to this *credibility* is that only one method of data collection was used. Although there may be justifiable reasons for this, it is generally considered that using other sources of data, for example observational data, focus group data or data from other similar studies, is a useful means by which to enhance the quality of qualitative studies (Spencer et al 2003). The use of other sources of data within a qualitative study to corroborate or indeed challenge initial findings is termed *triangulation* (Pope and Mays 2000).

Similar to May (2001), Sheppard et al (2010) also undertook individual face-to-face interviews but this was immediately following the encounter with the physiotherapist. Follow-up telephone interviews were conducted two to three weeks afterwards to enable further exploration in terms of the success of treatment or the appropriateness of onward referrals. The report by Sheppard et al (2010) briefly refers to the different data yielded from the different methods of interviews but did not *triangulate* the findings to corroborate or challenge the data collected using the different methods. Consideration of this, or at least reporting of it, would have offered a useful means to enhance the *credibility* of the findings (Pope and Mays 2000).

In contrast to the other two studies, Hills and Kitchen (2007) utilised individual interviews followed by focus groups, which are essentially facilitated group interviews. Focus groups can offer convenient means of seeking multiple view-points at one time and can be used to take advantage of a group dynamic where discussion and debate is stimulated by the responses of other group members, which is something that is missed during one-to-one interviews. In this study the individual interviews were used as a basis upon which to develop the topic guide for the focus group discussions, but the data generated from the focus groups is the core of this article. The authors reported that the study described in this article is part of a larger programme of research with the aim of developing a new satisfaction questionnaire. Although a common practice, for a variety of reasons, splitting of data is problematic for the reader who will subsequently need to find, review and then synthesise other articles to enable a full appraisal.

Although focus groups are commonly used in health services research, in our experience they can be difficult to organise and difficult to facilitate where commonly one or two dominant individuals lead the discussion and the other participants tend to follow their direction. Hills and Kitchen (2007) used four focus groups to collect data, with two of the groups consisting of patients defined as having acute musculoskeletal problems and two of the groups having chronic musculoskeletal problems. Using more than one focus group enabled these authors to contrast and hence *triangulate* their findings.

Despite different methods of data collection, one aspect that is common to all these studies is that physiotherapists conducted the interviews or focus groups. *Reflexivity* is a term commonly used within the qualitative literature to refer to the role of the researcher in generating data (Ritchie and Lewis 2003). Previously, whilst the quantitative paradigm was all dominant, some qualitative researchers would attempt to distance themselves from the process of data collection in an attempt to maintain neutrality or objectivity in keeping with features that are generally regarded as desirable within quantitative research. However, it is recognised that complete neutrality or objectivity when engaging with research participants is unrealistic. Instead a full and transparent report of the data collection process is preferred with the role of the researcher acknowledged.

Within the three included studies, it is not clear from the reports whether the researchers declared their backgrounds. It is generally recognised that most people try to please most of the time; so if a physiotherapist asks a question about physiotherapy it is likely that most people will try to please that physiotherapist by answering interview questions in a positive way. This environment might restrict the *credibility* of the responses, although May (2001) countered this by identifying that participants in his study did offer negative comments in relation to their experience. May (2001) was then able to use both positive and negative instances to generate the factors that underpin satisfaction. The fact that participants in all of these studies were recruited after they had experienced physiotherapy might safeguard against this threat to *credibility* because participants might not be concerned about whether their responses could affect their care since they had already been discharged. This could be more of an issue if participants were interviewed before they accessed physiotherapy. Sheppard et al (2010) reported the use of a reflexive diary but again do not report what this added to the process.

Data analysis

Unlike quantitative data analysis where there are clear and generally accepted guidelines, appraising the process of qualitative data analysis is not straightforward. There are two main reasons for this:

1) The multitude of different methods of data analysis,
2) The quality of the reporting of the data analysis process.

There is also significant overlap between methods of data analysis and it seems that different approaches are most often selected by researchers due to familiarity with the method rather than a robust argument in favour of one approach over the other.

The three included studies used framework analysis (May 2001), an interactive model of analysis (Hills and Kitchen 2007) and thematic analysis (Sheppard 2010). Due to the aforementioned difficulties and problems, in most cases, of justifying one approach over another it seems sensible to approach the appraisal of qualitative data analysis from a perspective of evaluating transparency and whether it is possible to see what has been undertaken and whether this is open to question. This enables a judgment regarding *confirmability*, which refers to whether the data collected supports the conclusions drawn.

Despite describing different methods of qualitative analysis, the three included papers all reported a very similar process of data collection followed by the identification and organisation of relevant themes from this data, for example, the personal and professional manner of the physiotherapist. May (2001) and Hills and Kitchen (2007) described how data analysis was undertaken by an individual and then verified by others. The process undertaken by Sheppard et al (2010) is unclear but the nature of the writing implies that this was undertaken by one individual. Vague reporting is a barrier to a useful critique and is a common problem across all types of research (Littlewood et al 2012b). The process undertaken by May (2001) and Hills and Kitchen (2007) is common in physiotherapy. Typically this work has been undertaken for educational reasons with no or little funding which precludes the use of other suitably qualified people to undertake independent data analysis. The limitations of a single person

Hills R and Kitchen S (2007). Satisfaction with outpatient physiotherapy: Focus groups to explore the views of patients with acute and chronic musculoskeletal conditions. Physiotherapy Theory and Practice, 23(1), 1-20.

Littlewood C, Ashton J, Mawson S, May S, Walters S (2012a). A mixed methods study to evaluate the clinical and cost-effectiveness of a self-managed exercise programme versus usual physiotherapy for chronic rotator cuff disorders: protocol for the SELF study. BMC Musculoskeletal Disorders, 13, 62.

Littlewood C, Ashton J, Chance-Larsen K, May S, Sturrock B (2012b). The quality of reporting might not reflect the quality of the study: implications for undertaking and appraising a systematic review. Journal of Manual and Manipulative Therapy, 20(3), 130-134.

Lincoln Y and Guba S (1985). Naturalistic Inquiry. Sage Publications, London, UK.

May S (2001). Patient satisfaction with management of back pain. Physiotherapy, 87(1), 4-20.

Petty N, Thomson O, Stew G (2012a). Ready for a paradigm shift? Part 1: Introducing qualitative research methodologies and methods. Manual Therapy, 17, 267-274.

Petty N, Thomson O, Stew G (2012b). Ready for a paradigm shift? Part 2: Introducing the philosophy of qualitative research. Manual Therapy, (In Press).

Pope C and Mays S (2000). Qualitative research in health care (2nd edition). BMJ publishing group; London, UK.

Ritchie J and Lewis J (2003). Qualitative research practice: a guide for social science students and researchers. Sage publications, London, UK.

Seale C (1999). The quality of qualitative research. Sage publications, London, UK.

Sheppard L, Anaf S, Gordon J (2010). Patient satisfaction with physiotherapy in the emergency department. International Emergency Nursing, 18, 196-202.

Spencer L, Ritchie J, Lewis J, Dillon L (2003). Quality in qualitative evaluation: a framework for assessing research evidence. Government Chief Social Researcher's Office, London, UK.

Author/ date/ title		
May (2001). An explorative, qualitative study into patients' satisfaction with physiotherapy.	Hills and Kitchen (2007). Satisfaction with outpatient physiotherapy: Focus groups to explore the views of patients with acute and chronic musculoskeletal conditions.	Sheppard et al (2010). Patient satisfaction with physiotherapy in the emergency department.
Research question/ aim		
To generate the range of dimensions of care that patients believe are important in their satisfaction with an episode of physiotherapy.	To explore the factors that affect patients' satisfaction with outpatient physiotherapy.	To explore patient satisfaction with emergency department (ED) physiotherapy.
Research design		
Qualitative	Qualitative	Qualitative
Sample/ context		
Purposive sample of patients who had received physiotherapy for low back pain in the previous year (n = 34). Community and district general hospital, UK.	Purposive sample of patients who had completed a course of outpatient physiotherapy in the previous four months (n = 30). Inner city and suburban hospitals, UK.	Purposive sample of adult patients who were treated by the ED physiotherapist during the period of on-site data collection (n = 22). Inner city ED, Australia.
Data Collection		
Individual face-to-face semi-structured interviews within the participants home, all conducted by a physiotherapy researcher.	Developmental interviews followed by focus groups, two comprising participants with acute musculoskeletal conditions (n = 4, n = 10) and two comprising participants with chronic musculoskeletal conditions (n = 5, n = 11), all conducted by a physiotherapy researcher.	Individual face-to-face semi-structured interviews (n = 22) within the ED followed by telephone interviews (n = 15), all conducted by a physiotherapy researcher.

Data analysis		
Framework analysis undertaken by one individual with verification by two other experienced qualitative researchers.	An interactive model of analysis was undertaken by one individual with verification by two other experienced physiotherapists.	Thematic analysis was undertaken by one individual.
Findings		
The main themes generated were: 1. Personal and professional manner of the therapist 2. Explanation as part of the treatment episode 3. Treatment as a consultative process 4. Access to care 5. Outcome.	The main themes generated were: 1. Expectations 2. Communications 3. Perceptions of the therapist 4. Treatment process 5. Outcome.	The main themes generated were: 1. Expectations 2. Bedside manner 3. Physiotherapy management 4. Satisfaction.

Table 3.1 Summary of included studies

CHAPTER FOUR

THE CASE STUDY OR CASE REPORT

Introduction

The case study or case report (different journals use different terms, but they mean the same thing), are non-experimental, observational reports from clinical practice. They present the case details of a single individual for their clinical and/or educational value. They can be used to describe an uncommon clinical presentation, a novel approach to diagnosis or a treatment that would not typically be administered. So, case studies can provide individual detail that is often missed in larger studies where groups of people are recruited. However because there is no control group in a case-study (discussed in chapter two and chapter eight), any observed change or treatment effect cannot be ascribed to the intervention with any confidence. Such observed changes could be explained simply by the passage of time including a concept known as regression to the mean, which refers to movement towards the average score over time. Alternatively, the placebo effect could explain any change. Furthermore the case study may not be generalisable beyond that individual and it is unlikely that such a report would make such a claim. However, this limitation is tempered by the detailed description of the case which is valuable for the reasons stated above.

Case studies or reports are commonly published in physiotherapy journals, hence their consideration in this book. The case studies to be appraised in this chapter are summarised in table 4.1 and it is recommended that you review these summaries before reading the forthcoming sections of this chapter.

Critical appraisal

The three case studies to be appraised are: Aina and May (2005), Littlewood and May (2007), and Menon and May (2012). There are no well-established or preferred quality criteria for case studies but the following account will consider components regarded as important by many. These criteria include an adequate description of the patient, use of appropriate outcome measures, and avoidance of accrediting causality to the intervention; meaning a direct suggestion that the treatment described was the sole factor explaining the clinical outcome should be avoided, due to the inherent limitations of the case study, as identified in the previous section.

Research aim and background

The three case studies clearly reported explicit aims relating to the intention to describe relatively novel clinical findings in the context of a case report. This enhances the *credibility* of the work and offers the reader some reassurance that the case study is an appropriate research design in this situation.

Descriptive detail

All of the case studies presented detail regarding age, gender, occupation as well as the findings from the history, including results from previous investigations, and the physical examination. Reporting of this detail facilitates *transferability* in terms of the reader being able to recognise patients with similar characteristics in their own clinics. However, only Menon and May (2012) reported their use of appropriate patient reported outcome measures. This is an important component which enhances the *credibility* of the case study because reliance is not placed on the authors of the case studies to report outcome, which might not actually be aligned with the opinion of the case/ patient.

Findings

Aina and May (2005) introduced the application of a therapeutic approach based upon a non-specific mechanical syndrome classification system. In keeping with the aim of a case study, this report was the first to offer this description in relation to mechanical diagnosis and therapy in the peer-reviewed literature. Whereas Aina and May (2005) described the application of repeated therapeutic movements, Littlewood and May (2007) introduced the application of loaded exercise based upon the same non-specific mechanical syndrome classification system. Both of these findings are in keeping with the role of a case study. Similarly Menon and May (2012) highlighted the potential benefits of a non-specific mechanical syndrome classification system in terms of the clinical assessment process compared to high-tech magnetic resonance imaging.

Implications and usefulness

Despite having value from an innovation and educational perspective, the case study offers limited opportunity to draw useful implications for clinical practice. Case studies are single patient-journey descriptions, and are selected for publication for some aspect of interest in that journey. Therefore there is obviously a huge potential for bias in this; for instance, was this patient commonplace or unique? We have no way of knowing. A consecutive-case series, which is simply multiple case studies collected with each relevant patient over a given period of time, is a better way of understanding if this was a normal or unusual clinical occurrence. But, whether a case study or a case-series, generalisability is always a problem. We can only speculate if this / these examples might relate to our patients in our clinics, which is clearly not an optimal foundation for evidence-based physiotherapy. Attempts at transferring the findings of a reported case study should be undertaken with a degree of caution due to the aforementioned limitations.

As a single case report we cannot know if changes in outcome were due to the intervention described in the report, or due to other factors, such as, placebo or natural history, which describes the fluctuations over time without intervention. As shown in the introduction case reports are not just about interventions but can be about, for instance, novel imaging reports being related to classification or clinical presentations. However if they do relate to interventions, as there is no control group, causality cannot be ascribed to the intervention described. These case reports may be useful building blocks to experimental trials, but cannot by themselves prove the worth of any intervention.

Summary

This chapter has introduced the case report and critically appraised three examples of this study design. The limitations of this study design have been identified, but also hopefully the reader can appreciate the potential usefulness of the case report to introduce novel ideas and to also serve as an educational tool.

References

Aina A and May S (2005). Case report – a shoulder derangement. Manual Therapy, 10, 159-163.

Littlewood C and May S (2007). A contractile dysfunction of the shoulder. Manual Therapy, 12, 80-83.

Menon A and May S (2012). Shoulder pain: differential diagnosis with mechanical diagnosis and therapy extremity assessment – a case report. Manual Therapy, (In Press).

The Case Study or Case Report

Author / date / title		
Aina and May (2005). Case report – a shoulder derangement.	Littlewood and May (2007). A contractile dysfunction of the shoulder.	Menon and May (2012). Shoulder pain: differential diagnosis with mechanical diagnosis and therapy assessment.
Research question / aim		
To describe a new method of assessment and management of shoulder pain using the principles of mechanical diagnosis and therapy.	To describe a new method of assessment and management of shoulder pain using the principles of mechanical diagnosis and therapy.	To describe a patient with shoulder pain who responded to repeated movements of the cervical spine using a mechanical diagnosis and therapy approach.
Research design		
Case report	Case report	Case report
Patient characteristics		
38-year old female physiotherapist.	57-year old male printer.	47-year old male technician.
Outcomes follow-up		
Asymptomatic at ten week follow-up.	Asymptomatic at ten week follow-up.	Asymptomatic at ten week follow-up.
Findings		
Patient was classified with derangement and repeated movements abolished symptoms and restored full movement at the shoulder in two sessions.	Patient was classified with contractile dysfunction and a programme of loaded abduction exercises abolished symptoms over ten weeks.	Patient was classified with cervical derangement, despite appearing to be a shoulder problem, and symptoms were abolished over four sessions.

Table 4.1 Summary of included studies

CHAPTER FIVE

CASE-CONTROL STUDY

Introduction

A case-control study is an observational study, in which two groups are compared; one group with a condition of interest or diagnosis and another matched group who do not have the condition of interest or diagnosis but are similar in other respects, for example in terms of age, gender, or occupation. The condition of interest or diagnosis could relate to a specific disease, specific clinical presentation, exposure to a particular risk, and so on. So, for instance, people with a specific clinical problem, such as back pain, could be compared with those who do not have back pain, and the frequency of different attributes could be compared, such as smoking, level of education, or physical conditions at work. In another example if a study showed 76% of men who had a heart attack drank alcohol, we would not know if alcohol was a risk factor for heart attack unless we could compare this group to men who had not had a heart attack, who would form the control group. In fact, what was found was that in those who had not had a heart attack 82% drank alcohol, and so alcohol was found to have a minor protective effect against heart attack (Crombie 1996).

The above examples highlight the most common use of the case-control study; to identify risk or protective factors for a specific condition or diagnosis. These studies tend to be retrospective in nature, which means looking back in time, or cross-sectional, which means at one point in time. So, typically the cases would be identified and recruited followed by recruitment of the matched controls (similar people in all aspects except for the condition of interest) before possible risk or protective actors are investigated through a review of clinical records, interviews or questionnaires.

As with every study design there are limitations and draw-backs. Remember, case-control studies cannot prove causation, only suggest an association, as highlighted in chapter two. Also, they are particularly susceptible to selection and recall bias. The potential for selection bias, resulting in systematic differences between the characteristics of the two groups, means that cases and controls have to be selected very carefully to

ensure, as far as possible, that the only difference between the two groups
was the presence or absence of the condition of interest or diagnosis.
Clearly, due to the complexity of human beings, this is an impossible task
and hence the potential for selection bias is always a threat to the validity
of case-control studies. Furthermore, as most case-control studies tend to
be retrospective, there is the potential problem of recall bias with past
events being plagued by memory loss and misremembering (Crombie
1996, Earl-Slater 2002).

The following section will offer a critical appraisal of three case-
control studies. The studies are summarised in table 5.1 and it is
recommended that you review these summaries before reading the
forthcoming sections of this chapter.

Critical appraisal

The three studies that have been selected for appraisal are: Womersley
and May (2006), Bakker et al (2007), May et al (2011), all of which
examined the effect of posture on low back pain.

Research question /aim

All three studies provided clear aims indicating their intention to
explore some link between postural or mechanical loads and back pain.
Two of the studies (Womersley and May 2006, May et al 2011)
investigated McKenzie's postural syndrome; a specific classification of
low back pain, whereas the other investigated the role of postural loading
on back pain in general (Bakker et al 2007).

Research design

All of the studies investigated risk factors for some type of low back
pain. As identified earlier, this is a bona fide research question to ask
using a case-control study design. Two of the studies used a cross-
sectional data collection method with the use of a questionnaire (Bakker et
al 2007) or a questionnaire and a physical examination (May et al 2011).
The other study collected data over a three day period as well as
comparing cases and controls with a physical examination at the end of
this period (Womersley and May 2006). All studies had a structured way
of contrasting those with and without back pain.

Sample

All three studies used a non-randomised voluntary recruitment process from a specific population, either a student or general practice setting. A randomised recruitment process is not appropriate for case-control studies as there is a specific requirement to recruit those with and without a problem, in this case back pain, and then to compare these groups. In some ways this is similar to the purposive recruitment process described in chapter three for qualitative studies, but here a control group is also needed who are as similar as possible to the case group except for the condition of interest or diagnosis, in this situation low back pain.

The case group was identified in all studies as those with some sort of non-specific low back pain. Operational definitions were provided in two studies (Womersley and May 2006, May et al 2011) which enables the reader to clearly identify the nature of the complaints of the participants who were included. The control group was recruited from the same setting in all studies and comparison was undertaken using questionnaires and physical examinations on certain postural variables including length of time sitting, degree of flexion when sitting etc. Statistical analysis was conducted between the cases and controls on these variables to identify true differences. As with all study designs, external validity or generalisability is an issue. However, we do know who the participants were with regards to age, gender, and other variables, which provides the reader with sufficient information to adequately consider issues of relevance and external validity.

Only one study provided a sample-size calculation and recruited what would be regarded as a large sample size for each group (Bakker et al 2007). One reason for conducting a sample-size calculation is to estimate the number of participants required to detect a difference between the study groups, if one really exists. If a study recruits too few participants, this might result in a Type II error which is said to have occurred if a study fails to identify a difference between the study groups that actually exists in reality. However, despite small sample sizes in the other two studies, statistically significant differences were found between cases and controls, indicating that a Type II error was not an issue.

Data collection

The data collection methods varied between the studies, but depended upon the specific research questions being addressed. Studies used self-report questionnaires (Womersley and May 2006), clinician-reported questionnaires (Bakker et al 2007, May et al 2011), or physical examination or computerised video analysis (Womersley and May 2006, May et al 2011), all of which were relevant to the research questions being asked. The studies used established data collection methods, or made an attempt to establish the validity or reliability of the data collection methods. Data collection methods may need to be created to address specific novel research questions. If so it is important that some attempt is made to establish the *trustworthiness* of these methods, as was done here which enhances the *credibility* of the studies.

Data analysis

In all three studies the cases and controls were compared statistically on certain variables to establish if there was a difference beyond what would be expected by chance. In all studies p-values indicated statistically significant differences between the group with back pain and those without, so we can be reasonably certain that these differences were unlikely to be due to chance. Bakker et al (2007) also conducted what is known as a multivariate regression analysis. This is a more sophisticated method of analysis, in which the strength of the different variables associated with back pain were compared with each other to see which ones were most important. This type of analysis is very useful when a number of factors might indicate a risk for a particular outcome, as the strengths of risk are compared to see which is strongest.

The studies used different statistical tests to compare the cases and the controls. The tests used depended on the type of data that was being collected and tested (see glossary). The preferred method for case-control studies is to report the degree of risk with which a factor might be associated with a particular outcome (Altman 1991). This is done with odds ratios, which was used by Bakker et al (2007) or relative risks. These are interpreted as one, meaning the risks are the same for both groups, or less than or greater than one, meaning one of the groups has a greater risk for that outcome. The further away from one then the greater the risk is. Bakker et al (2007) found that with more sustained flexed postures the odds ratio for back pain was 1.4 to 2.7 depending on time. In other words the risk of back pain increased the more these postures were maintained, which again suggests a level of certainty about this link.

Findings

The main methods used and the findings are summarised in table 5.1. Despite the different contexts in which the studies were conducted and the difference in research methods and data analysis, some similarities between the findings of the studies are evident. All supported an association between non-specific low back pain and posture in clinical and non-health care seeking populations. In these studies sustained sitting and more flexed postures were consistently associated with greater risk of low back pain.

Implications and usefulness

Despite some limitations in the included studies and their different methodologies, they all offer a useful insight into factors, namely sustained sitting and flexed postures, which were consistently found to be associated with back pain. As stated in the introduction, association is not the same as causation which cannot be implied here. Together these studies have highlighted a potential link between posture and low back pain but to be clear, they do not prove that poor posture causes low back pain. Indeed it is possible that low back pain might contribute to the development of poor postures or that posture is associated with another factor, for example work-load stress, that might cause low back pain. Hence from these case-control studies it is not clear whether postural education might be a useful component of evidence-based physiotherapy.

Summary

This chapter has introduced the case-control study design. The common methodology has been described and three published case-control studies have been critically appraised. The studies varied from a large multi-centre context to relatively small single-centre context, and from relatively straightforward to more complex data analysis, but all considered risk factors or association between risk factors and non-specific low back pain. The chapter has offered readers a basis upon which to approach and critically appraise the work of others and/or begin to develop their own study.

References

Altman D (1991). Practical Statistics for Medical Research. Chapman and Hall, London.
Bakker E, Verhagen A, Lucas C, Koning H, de Hann R, Koes B (2007). Daily spinal mechanical loading as a risk factor for acute non-specific

low back pain: a case-control study using the 24-Hour Schedule. European Spine Journal, 16, 107-113.

Crombie I (1996). Research in Healthcare. Design, Conduct and Interpretation of Health Services Research. John Wiley and Sons, Chichester.

Earl-Slater A (2002). The Handbook of Clinical Trials and Other Research. Radcliffe Medical Press, Oxford.

May S, Nanche G, Pingle S (2011). High frequency of McKenzie's postural syndrome in young population of non-care seeking individuals. Journal of Manual and Manipulative Therapy, 19, 48-54.

Womersley L and May S (2006). Sitting posture of subjects with postural backache. Journal of Manual and Manipulative Therapy, 29, 213-218.

Author / date / title		
Womersley and May (2006). Sitting posture of subjects with postural backache.	Bakker et al (2007). Daily spinal loading as a risk factor for acute non-specific low back pain: a case-control study using the 24-Hour Schedule.	May et al (2011). High Frequency of McKenzie's postural syndrome in young population of non-care seeking individuals.
Research question / aim		
To determine if sitting periods and flexed relaxed sitting postures were risk factors for postural backache.	To assess spinal mechanical loading as potential independent risk factors for acute back pain.	To assess risk factors for those reporting possible postural backache.
Research design		
Case-control with prospective data collection over three day period.	Case-control with prospective data collection over 24-hour period.	Two stage case-control with cross-sectional data collection.
Sample / context		
Student volunteers: postural backache group (N = 9), and non-postural backache group (N = 9). Two groups similar in age, gender-mix, height and weight.	Patients attending GP clinic with acute episode of back pain (N = 100); attending GP clinical for another problem, but no back pain for at least 12 months (N = 100). No significant differences in outcomes at baseline; very similar in age, gender-mix, weight, and height.	66 with possible postural backache; three with backache with other classification; 31 no history of backache. Baseline data not given for the two groups. 37 / 66 agreed to physical examination: 31 / 37 confirmed with postural syndrome.
Data collection		
Use of self-completed activity diary over three days; then computerised video recording of posture after ten minutes of relaxed sitting.	Physiotherapists performed questionnaires at baseline and 24 hours.	Face-to-face recruitment and use of questionnaire; then standard McKenzie assessment.

Data analysis		
Mann Whitney U test to identify differences between cases and controls.	Odds ratios presented to identify which postures were associated with backache compared to the controls. Odds ratio of $\geq$ 1.5 considered clinically relevant; multivariate analysis to confirm importance of significant variables.	Correlation coefficients used to identify factors that were associated with McKenzie's postural syndrome.
Findings		
There were 46 backache episodes in the backache group, but none in the control group. Those in the backache group sat for longer periods without interruption, and their relaxed sitting posture was more flexed.	The backache group were more likely to use postures of flexion than the controls, who were more likely to use extended postures.	In those with suspected and proven postural syndrome sustained sitting was the commonest cause.

Table 5.1 Summary of included studies

CHAPTER SIX

COHORT STUDY

Introduction

A cohort study is an observational study in which a particular group, with some shared characteristic, is observed. Cohort studies are regarded as longitudinal studies because outcomes, for example the presence or absence of knee pain, are collected over time. Probably the most influential cohort study was that conducted by Doll et al (1964, 1976, 1994, 2004). This study recruited 40 000 male doctors, allocated them into four cohorts and followed them up over 50 years. The cohorts (shared characteristics) were non-smokers, and light, moderate and heavy smokers with death as the outcome. Impressively the authors managed to collect data from 94% of living participants over the long-term. The study showed a substantially higher lung cancer and all-causes of mortality in the smokers, with a dose-response relationship, that is the more you smoked the greater chance of mortality. This study went a long way to demonstrate that the link between smoking and death might be causal and not coincidental (Greenhalgh 2010).

Most commonly cohort studies are prospective, meaning that outcomes are collected from a certain time point forwards. A minority of cohort studies are retrospective or looking back over time. Cohort studies are most commonly used to explore the natural history of a condition, risk factors and/ or prognostic factors. For instance a systematic review of cohort studies looked at who was likely to develop neck pain (McLean et al 2010). Fourteen cohort studies were located, in which participants were free of pain at the start and then followed up for one year. The presence or absence of neck pain was recorded over time. Several risk factors for the development of neck pain were identified including; female gender, older age, high job demands, being an ex-smoker, and history of previous back or neck pain (McLean et al 2010).

Another systematic review of cohort studies investigated factors that might impact upon prognosis by retrieving studies that had recruited people with neck pain at the outset (McLean et al 2007). Several prognostic factors were associated with poor outcomes including; older age, longer duration of symptoms, a previous history of neck pain, and co-existing shoulder or other musculoskeletal problems. Interestingly, regular exercise strongly predicted a good outcome.

A possible source of bias is loss to follow-up, which means that outcome data, for example presence or absence of knee pain or functional status or quality of life, has not been collected from research participants. Loss to follow-up is common in research studies for a variety of reasons including participants moving house without notifying the research team so they are no longer contactable; some participants may die, particularly if the follow-up is over a long period of time, or participants might become disaffected and not want to engage with the research study anymore. Loss to follow-up is common in all research studies and it is recognised that achieving 100% follow-up, even in the short-term, is highly unlikely. Most studies will expect to lose between 15 to 20% of their participants over time, more if the follow-up period is greater than one year (Hudak et al 1996) and will set out to recruit more participants from the outset, if possible, to account for this loss. Why is this a source of bias though? Well, if we don't have data about people we don't know anything about them. It is possible that the participants who drop-out and hence become lost to follow-up are different in some way to those who don't drop-out and so any conclusions we draw are susceptible to bias. In the context of a cohort study, if a higher proportion of research participants with lower socioeconomic status drop-out, the capacity to draw conclusions about this group is limited. In the context of a randomised controlled trial, drop-out might be related to the experience of the interventional treatment. So, consider if all the participants who had a negative response to a treatment dropped-out; this would mean that most of the participants remaining in the group would report a positive response which is not reflective of the truth and serves to inflate the reported effect of an intervention.

A range of opinion exists regarding the factors that should be considered when appraising observational cohort studies (Hayden et al 2006). Important factors to consider include whether the study sample was representative of the population of interest, loss to follow-up, adequate measurement of risk and prognostic factors and outcomes along with consideration of whether statistical analysis was appropriate.

With these considerations in mind, the following section will offer a critical appraisal of three cohort studies. The studies are summarised in table 6.1 and it is recommended that you review these summaries before reading the forthcoming sections of this chapter.

Critical appraisal

The three studies that have been selected for review considered whether a phenomenon known as centralization could predict outcome in people with back pain and/ or sciatica (Werneke et al 1999, Werneke and Hart 2001, Skytte et al 2005). Centralization refers to a situation where pain thought to be of spinal origin moves from a distal, for example the leg, to a more proximal location, for example the back, in response to a specific movement or therapeutic loading strategy, for example repeated lumbar flexion, before the back pain is abolished.

Research design

All studies were prospective cohort studies. One study followed patients only to discharge (Werneke et al 1999), the other two followed patients up for one year, with one a long-term follow-up from the previous cohort (Werneke and Hart 2001). Knowing the long-term outcomes a one-year follow-up is most useful in a condition like low back pain that is known to be frequently persistent or chronic.

Sample

In the first study (Werneke et al 1999) the patients had back or neck pain of less than six weeks duration, so a clearly defined group were recruited to allow the reader to judge the applicability of the findings to their own population. Two hundred and twenty three patients with back pain were tracked over the year after discharge in the second part of the study (Werneke and Hart 2001). In the other study patients were recruited with sub-acute sciatica; so again a clearly defined population was included to allow readers to understand who this population was (Skytte et al 2005). From the demographic details provided we can be reasonably confident that these patients were similar to other patients with these symptoms regarding age, gender, area of symptoms, duration of symptoms, work status etc. Because of the potential bias caused by loss to follow-up it has been suggested that an 85% follow-up rate is adequate, but obviously there is something rather arbitrary about this percentage rate. So the 84% follow-up in one paper (Werneke and Hart 2001), and over 85% in the other paper (Skytte et al 2005) would be regarded as more than adequate by most.

Data collection

The person undertaking data collection in all of these studies was blinded, meaning unaware, to patient demographics, response to treatment and centralization status. Blinding here reduces the risk of bias because any pre-conceived thoughts or ideas that the data collector might have are not allowed to influence this process. For example, if the data collector was keen to prove the value of centralization and knew whether the patients had demonstrated centralization or not, they might be more inclined to report favourably in relation to this group.

Baseline data was collected in two studies (Werneke et al 1999, Skytte et al 2005), and follow-up data at one-year, and at two and six months and one year in two studies (Werneke and Hart 2001, Skytte et al. 2005). Baseline data reported in Werneke and Hart (2001) included demographic and historical variables, job factors, psychosocial factors, rehabilitation programme factors and centralization status. Outcomes were pain severity, return to work, sick leave from work, activity interference at home, and continued use of healthcare. Baseline data reported in Skytte et al (2005) were pain and disability measures, sick leave, demographic data, beliefs about return to work, nature of symptoms, and centralization status, and outcome data were pain, disability, and spine surgery. The baseline data not only allows the reader to get an understanding of the patient group, but also includes some psychosocial factors that other studies have suggested are important determinants of long-term outcome. To restrict baseline data to centralization status only would possibly exaggerate its importance and downplay the role of those other factors. The outcomes reflect a range of measures that are important from a societal perspective as they include work status, further care and surgery, which all have cost implications.

Data analysis

Whereas Werneke et al (1999) did not present a multivariate regression analysis, Werneke and Hart (2001) and Skytte et al (2005) did. This type of analysis is important as it seeks to consider the relative importance of the factors just mentioned against each other. In other words it allows the reader to judge if centralization-status was a less or more important predictor of long-term outcome than the psychosocial factors. It does this by individually evaluating which factors predicted the outcomes, in a so-called univariate analysis. Then it compares the significant predictors with each other to see which is the strongest predictor, in a so-called multivariate analysis. This type of analysis is very appropriate in a cohort study as it includes multiple potentially important predictors, and compares them against each other.

Findings

In the first paper there were significant differences in pain and disability outcomes between the centralization and partial centralization groups and the non-centralization group (Werneke et al 1999). At one year, nine of the 23 variables affected one or more outcomes in the univariate analysis, with perceived disability at discharge, centralization status, and overt pain behaviour affecting outcomes most commonly. In the multivariate analysis centralization status affected pain (p=0.004), return to work (p<0.001), activity interference (p<0.001), and healthcare use (p<0.001), and leg pain at intake affected sick leave (p=0.004) (Werneke and Hart 2001). In other words centralization was a stronger predictor of outcome than any of the other variables that were included. Because the p-values are small these findings were highly unlikely to be a chance finding.

In patients with sciatica centralization at baseline was associated with better outcomes at several time points, and even at one year in terms of pain and disability, and patients with non-centralization at baseline were six times more likely to end up undergoing spinal surgery (Skytte et al 2005). Both studies thus attest to the importance of this clinical finding in terms predicting a good outcome if centralization was present, and a poor outcome if centralization was not present.

Implications and usefulness

Clinically there are a number of implications that arise from these studies. Centralization has positive prognostic implications for neck pain short-term, and for back pain and sciatica short and long-term. Conversely non-centralization is associated with a poor prognosis. These findings might be different in different populations but these studies used clearly defined patient groups, collected data on a range of important factors at baseline, followed up for one year a sizeable proportion of all patients, and looked at a range of important healthcare outcomes.

Summary

This chapter has introduced the cohort study design, described their advantages for studies into risk and prognostic factors and also highlighted aspects of the methodology to be aware of when reading such studies. A critique of three studies has also been offered against some specific criteria that will allow readers to critically appraise other cohort studies. This introductory platform enables consideration of the usefulness of cohort studies to inform clinical practice.

References

Doll R and Hill A (1964). Mortality in relation to smoking: 10 years' observations on British doctors. British Medical Journal, I, 1399-1467.

Doll R and Peto R (1976). Mortality in relation to smoking: 20 years' observations on British doctors. British Medical Journal, I, 1525-1536.

Doll R, Peto R, Wheatley K, Gray R (1994). Mortality in relation to smoking: 40 years' observations on British doctors. British Medical Journal, 309, 901-911.

Doll R, Peto R, Boreham J, Sutherland I (2004). Mortality in relation to smoking: 50 years' observations on British doctors. British Medical Journal, 328, 1519-1528.

Greenhalgh T (2010). How to read a paper (4th edition). Wiley-Blackwell, Chichester,UK.

Hayden J, Cote P, Bombardier C (2006). Evaluation of the quality of prognosis studies in systematic reviews. Annals of Internal Medicine, 144(6), 427-37.

Hudak P, Cole D, Haines A (1996). Understanding prognosis to improve rehabilitation: the example of lateral elbow pain. Archives of Physical Medicine and Rehabilitation, 77, 586-593.

McLean S, May S, Klaber-Moffett J, Sharp, D, Gardner E (2007). Prognostic factors for progressive non-specific neck pain: a systematic review. Physical Therapy Reviews, 12, 207-220.

McLean S, May S, Klaber-Moffett J, Sharp D, Gardiner E (2010). Risk factors for the onset of non-specific neck pain: a systematic review. Journal of Epidemiology and Community Health, 64, 565-572.

Skytte L, May S, Petersen P (2005). Centralization: its prognostic value in patients with referred symptoms and sciatica. Spine, 30, E293-E299.

Werneke M, Hart D, Cook D (1999). A descriptive study of the centralization phenomenon. A prospective analysis. Spine, 24, 676-683.

Werneke M and Hart D (2001). Centralization phenomenon as a prognostic factor for chronic low back pain and disability. Spine, 26, 758-765.

Cohort Study

Author / date / title		
Werneke et al (1999) A descriptive study of the centralization phenomenon. A prospective analysis.	Werneke and Hart (2001). Centralization phenomenon as a prognostic factor for chronic low back pain and disability.	Skytte et al (2005). Centralization: its prognostic value in patients with referred symptoms and sciatica.
Research question / aim		
To standardise operational definition of centralization; to determine prevalence according to this definition; to evaluate reliability; to determine outcomes in different groups.	To evaluate using a range of baseline variables (demographic, work-related, psychosocial, centralization status) on long-term outcome.	To determine prognostic significance of centralization-status at baseline on long-term outcomes, including surgical status.
Research design		
A prospective analysis of occurrence and outcomes in a cohort.	Long-term (1 year) follow-up of previous cohort (Werneke et al 1999).	A prospective, comparative cohort study with 1 year follow-up.
Sample		
351 patients with acute (< 6 weeks) neck or back pain.	223 patients with back pain at baseline (patients with neck pain excluded).	60 patients referred for suspected disc herniation with referred symptoms.
Data collection		
Centralization (31%), partial centralization (46%) and non-centralization (23%) groups compared at discharge on pain, disability and treatment visits.	Status evaluated 1 year after discharge from physical therapy between centralization and non-centralization on pain, work status, disability and health care use.	Centralization (25) and non-centralization (35) status determined at baseline and groups compared at different time points for pain, disability and surgery.
Data analysis		
Analysis of variance for differences in outcome between groups.	Univariate analysis of baseline factors' predictive value at long-term; multivariate analysis of significant factors.	Analysis of variance for differences in outcome between groups.

Findings
Differences in number of visits (3.9, 8.0, 7.7 respectively) (p<0.001), and centralization / partial centralization versus non-centralization.	9 / 23 variables affected outcomes long-term; only centralization status (pain, p=0.004; work status, disability, use of health care p<0.001) and leg pain at intake (sick leave, p=0.004) remained significant.	Differences in leg pain (p<0.05 at 2, 3months), back pain (p<0.05 at 3 months), and disability (p<0.05 at 1, 2, 3,12 months); more surgery in non-centralization group (p=0.01), odds ratio 6.2.

Table 6.1 Summary of included studies

CHAPTER SEVEN

CROSS-SECTIONAL STUDY

Introduction

Cross-sectional is a broad term that could be used to describe a variety of studies. Whereas longitudinal studies, for example the cohort study (described in chapter six), collect data over time, the cross-sectional study collects data at one point in time (Herbert et al 2005). In physiotherapy, the term cross-sectional study can be applied to studies investigating the number of people complaining of a certain problem or disease, surveys of current practice and studies of diagnostic accuracy. In the first example, a snapshot is taken to understand the extent of a problem and in the second example, a survey of current practice enables an understanding of how a clinical problem is currently treated and/or how treatment has changed in response to, for example, publication of treatment guidelines. The third example, the diagnostic accuracy study, enables an understanding of how one or a group of clinical tests, for example the straight leg raise, compares to a gold or reference standard test, for example magnetic resonance imaging, when making a diagnosis. Another common type of cross-sectional study, conducted in physiotherapy in relation to the accuracy of clinical tests, is the reliability study. In these, two or more therapists are compared to see if they reach the same conclusion when using a specific test. For instance, if when using a McMurray's test do the therapists agree if the patient has a meniscal injury or not?

The following section will offer a critical appraisal of three cross-sectional studies. The first relates to a study that investigated the point prevalence of shoulder tendinitis (Frost et al 2002), i.e. the number of people with shoulder tendinitis at one point in time (Harris and Taylor 2004), the second is a survey of current practice (Littlewood et al 2012) and the third is a diagnostic accuracy study (Kelly et al 2010) that has direct relevance to the findings of the survey. The studies are summarised in table 7.1 and it is recommended that you review these summaries before reading the forthcoming sections of this chapter.

Critical appraisal

As has already been mentioned, and will be mentioned again, a range of tools are available to aid the process of critical appraisal. Again, we will cover features regarded as being important in studies of this nature, but specifically for readers interested in developing their understanding of quality appraisal of diagnostic accuracy studies beyond this chapter we recommend Whiting et al (2011) as a starting point.

Research question/ aim

Among other aims, Frost et al (2002) provided a clear statement regarding their intention to report prevalence of shoulder tendinitis. Littlewood et al (2012) clearly aimed to describe current practice in relation to the assessment and management of rotator cuff disorders whereas Kelly et al (2010) aimed to determine the diagnostic accuracy of commonly used physical tests for subacromial impingement syndrome using diagnostic ultrasound as the reference standard.

Research design

The aim of all three studies clearly aligned with the accepted role of cross-sectional studies. Despite this, it is important to recognise some inherent limitations of the cross-sectional design. For example, with reference to Littlewood et al (2012), even if we accept the findings of the survey of current practice, they are just that; findings at that point in time. It is highly possible that clinical practice will change in response to publication of research and clinical practice guidelines over time and hence such findings might be quickly outdated. Many would suggest that such a speedy change in clinical practice is somewhat optimistic but it should be borne in mind. So, what is the point in undertaking a cross-sectional study of this nature? Well, it does provide us with an important understanding of practice at a point in time which enables future studies to evaluate whether practice is changing or responding to the best available evidence over time.

With reference to Kelly et al (2010), their participants were exposed to a range of clinical tests, which were defined as being either positive or negative, before undergoing a diagnostic ultrasound scan. This is a common design in cross-sectional diagnostic accuracy studies where the capacity of one or a range of tests is compared to the gold or reference standard test; which in this situation is diagnostic ultrasound. In simplistic terms the gold or reference-standard test is the test which is regarded as being capable of giving the "correct" diagnosis, in this case subacromial impingement syndrome. Sometimes the term validity is applied to studies of this nature where the aim is to establish whether the clinical test can determine the truth with reference to the gold standard. Usually the reference-standard tests are more time consuming, more costly and less accessible; other common examples of such tests include magnetic resonance imaging or surgical findings. So, if a less expensive, less time-consuming and more accessible test can be found that still enables a diagnosis to be formulated with acceptable accuracy in comparison to the reference test, then it would clearly be preferable. Hopefully it will be apparent to you that the reference-standard test used is a key quality feature of a cross-sectional diagnostic accuracy study. If a sub-standard test, i.e. a test that cannot accurately diagnose the condition, is used, then clearly comparison against it will also be sub-standard and will be of limited clinical value. Frequently the authors will justify the use of their reference-standard test, as Kelly et al (2010) did; from the perspective of accuracy but also that it can be performed within a time frame where the clinical condition is likely to remain unaltered. One concern with diagnostic accuracy studies is that the clinical test is performed and then there is a delay before the reference test is performed, particularly if this is a surgical-reference test. This means that the clinical condition could change during the testing intervals and so the clinical and then reference test would actually be examining different things which clearly would invalidate any attempt to determine diagnostic accuracy. If the justification for the reference test is not reported then it would be wise to investigate this further through a review of the relevant literature. In this case, diagnostic ultrasound is regarded as an appropriate reference standard by many, but this is open to challenge. It is becoming increasingly apparent, because identified structural pathology is not strongly associated with clinical signs and symptoms, that it is wholly inappropriate to judge these clinical tests against reference tests which aim to identify structural pathology. For example, Frost et al (1999) were unable to differentiate between individuals diagnosed with subacromial impingement and asymptomatic age-matched controls according to structural pathology. Hence, such reference tests are of limited clinical use when employed in this manner because it is irrelevant whether the clinical test can identify the structural pathology because the pathology is likely to be irrelevant also. What is the point in using a test that identifies irrelevant findings accurately? A more appropriate research design for diagnostic accuracy studies might begin with tests that enable a judgement about the appropriate treatment to be offered; which in turn results in a good treatment outcome which is regarded as the gold standard, rather than a test of dubious value. Hence, there is probably more of a useful role for longitudinal diagnostic accuracy studies rather than cross-sectional in situations where the diagnosis generated by the gold or reference standard does not usefully inform treatment or predict outcome. Such longitudinal design could easily be embedded within randomised controlled trials, discussed in chapter eight.

Sample/ context

Frost et al (2002) clearly defined their study sample such that it would be possible to identify similar patients in clinical practice; this is a clear strength which aids generalisability as does the fact that they drew their sample from a relatively large group of working adults. However, only 66% of the participants initially approached subsequently responded to the questionnaires and then underwent a physical examination to confirm the diagnosis of shoulder tendinitis. The concern here is that the numbers involved might not sufficiently represent the wider population which, despite the above points, introduces some uncertainty about the generalisability of the findings.

Littlewood et al (2012) recruited 110 physiotherapists with experience of treating rotator cuff disorders. The respondents had a wide variety of experience and reported a range of practice settings. Fifty of the respondents reported having a special interest in rotator cuff disorders whereas 60 did not. The wide range of respondents in terms of experience, practice setting and special interest is useful to characterise the range of practice that is undertaken but considering the number of physiotherapists in the UK, a sample of 110 might not be regarded as being capable of providing findings that are generalisable to the wider population.

Kelly et al (2010) recruited participants who had been referred for diagnostic ultrasonography as part of a usual clinical pathway. This is useful from a generalisability perspective. However, only 34 patient participants were recruited and only one physiotherapist performed the clinical tests and only one radiologist performed the ultrasound scans. Again, the number of participants is relatively small and only having one physiotherapist and one radiologist performing the tests minimises the variability in testing which means that the results are likely to be overly optimistic. More variability and uncertainty would be introduced if a wider range of clinicians were performing the tests which would more than likely impact upon the diagnostic accuracy.

Data collection

When considering the aims of these studies, the methods of data collection appear suitable. Specifically, other methods, for example individual interviews, were potentially open to Littlewood et al (2012) but the time requirement would prohibit the collection of large amounts of data.

One concern with diagnostic accuracy studies is whether the results of one test are interpreted in the knowledge of the results of the other test. So, the clinical tests suggest a positive diagnosis and this is known to the person performing the reference test; do you think this could influence their interpretation of the output of the reference test? The answer recognised by most is yes! However, Kelly et al (2010) overcame this design flaw by structuring the study so that the reference test was completed first and then the physiotherapist undertaking the clinical tests was blinded to the results meaning that they were unaware of the reference test results. This enhances the internal validity of this study meaning that we can trust the findings to a greater degree than if the physiotherapist had not been blinded to the results.

Data analysis

In comparison to some other studies, the statistics used here are relatively straightforward. Both Frost et al (2002) and Littlewood et al (2012) were largely looking to describe and summarise their data and so descriptive statistics were appropriately employed. Littlewood et al (2012) also used the Chi-squared test to determine whether the responses of those regarding themselves as having a special interest in rotator cuff disorders compared to those who did not was significantly different. This is an appropriate statistic in this context (Harris and Taylor 2004) and, among other results, showed that physiotherapists who regarded themselves as having a special interest were employed in more senior roles.

Kelly et al (2010) reported sensitivity, specificity, likelihood ratios and overall accuracy for each physical examination test. Although these statistics are not immediately intuitive or easy to remember, reference to any statistics book for a quick refresher, for example Harris and Taylor (2004), will reassure you that these were appropriate. In this context, sensitivity refers to the proportion of participants with subacromial impingement syndrome defined by the ultrasound scan that also had a positive result with the physical examination test. Specificity refers to the proportion of participants without subacromial impingement syndrome defined by the ultrasound scan that also had a negative result with the physical examination test. Likelihood ratios refer to the likelihood of the test being positive in those with subacromial impingement syndrome defined by the ultrasound scan compared to those who were negative to the scan. Nowadays this is the preferred way to report this type of data because it uses all the data, both those who were positive to the scan and those who were negative.

Findings

Frost et al (2002) reported the point prevalence of shoulder tendinitis as 3.2% which indicates a relatively common musculoskeletal complaint. Littlewood et al (2012) reported that the respondents to the survey of current practice would undertake a wide range of diagnostic tests, offer a wide variety of treatment and offer a broad prediction of prognosis. Advice and exercise were the most common prescriptions which appears to be largely justified with reference to current literature although the type and dose remain unclear. Many of the other suggested interventions however are not supported by current evidence (Littlewood et al 2012). Finally, Kelly et al (2010) suggested that the physical examination tests evaluated in their study have limited capacity to inform diagnosis when compared to diagnostic ultrasound as the reference standard.

Implications and usefulness

The implications of Frost et al (2002) are that shoulder tendinitis, as they define it, is a relatively common musculoskeletal condition which clearly deserves attention from clinicians, researchers and commissioners. Littlewood et al (2012) highlighted the range of current practice which enables a judgement about the extent to which current best evidence is translated into clinical practice but also offers a foundation upon which the impact of future research and clinical guidelines can be evaluated. It seems reasonable to suggest that both of these studies have greater research implications and are more useful in this context rather than to the individual physiotherapist. However, the study by Kelly et al (2012) has implications for both clinical and research practice. Notwithstanding the limitations of using diagnostic ultrasound in the context of cross-sectional diagnostic accuracy studies, much of clinical practice remains based upon a biomedical model where identification of structural pathology as a basis for explaining pain remains. The study by Kelly et al (2010) reiterates the work of others which demonstrates that commonly used physical examination tests have limited predictive value in this context. Hence, such research should serve as a stimulus for physiotherapists to challenge what should now be regarded as outdated practice.

Summary

This chapter has introduced a range of studies that are commonly described under the cross-sectional umbrella. Three published studies have been described and critically appraised before the implications and usefulness of the studies for clinical and research practice have been considered. The critical appraisal has recognised the limitations of this research design and hence has offered a basis upon which the novice researcher can approach and critically appraise other similar studies.

References

Frost P, Andersen J, Lundorf E (1999). Is supraspinatus pathology as defined by magnetic resonance impaging associated with clinical signs of shoulder impingement? Journal of Shoulder and Elbow Surgery, 8, 565-568.

Frost P, Bonder J, Mikkelsen S, Andersen J, Fallentin N, Kaergaard A, Thomsen J (2002). Risk of shoulder tendinitis in relation to shoulder loads in monotonous repetitive work. American Journal of Industrial Medicine, 41, 11-18.

Harris M and Taylor G (2004). Medical Statistics Made Easy. Thomson Publishing Services, UK.

Herbert R, Jamtvedt G, Mead J, Hagen K (2005). Practical Evidence-Based Physiotherapy. Elsevier, UK.

Kelly S, Brittle N, Allen G (2010). The value of physical tests for subacromial impingement syndrome: a study of diagnostic accuracy. Clinical rehabilitation, 24, 149-158.

Littlewood C, Lowe A, Moore J (2012). Rotator cuff disorders: a survey of current UK physiotherapy practice. Shoulder and Elbow, 4(1), 64-71.

Whiting P, Rutjes A, Westwood M, Mallett S, Deeks J, Reitsma J, Leeflang M, Sterne J, Bossuyt P, and the QUADAS-2 Group (2011). QUADAS-2: A Revised Tool for the Quality Assessment of Diagnostic Accuracy Studies. Annals of Internal Medicine, 155, 529-536.

Author/ date/ title		
Frost et al (2002). Risk of shoulder tendinitis in relation to shoulder loads in monotonous repetitive work.	Littlewood et al (2012). Rotator cuff disorders: a survey of current UK physiotherapy practice.	Kelly et al (2010). The value of physical tests for subacromial impingement syndrome: a study of diagnostic accuracy.
Research question/ aim		
To describe point prevalence of shoulder tendinitis.	To describe current practice in relation to the assessment and management of rotator cuff disorders.	To determine the diagnostic accuracy of physical tests for subacromial impingement syndrome.
Research design		
Cross-sectional	Cross-sectional survey	Cross-sectional/ diagnostic accuracy
Sample		
4 162 Danish workers were invited to participate. Shoulder tendinitis was defined as; shoulder pain provoked with movement against resistance or positive impingement sign.	110 physiotherapists with experience of treating rotator cuff disorders.	Thirty-four patients, median age 57 years, 20 (59%) male, referred for diagnostic ultrasonography complaining of shoulder pain of > 4 months duration. One physiotherapist undertook the physical examination screening and one consultant radiologist performed the diagnostic ultrasound evaluation.

Data Collection		
Questionnaire regarding presence of shoulder symptoms followed by a physical examination to confirm diagnosis.

Of the 4 162 who were invited to participate, 3 123 returned the questionnaires and 2 743 (66%) underwent physical examination to confirm diagnosis. | An online survey distributed via professional networks. | The report of the ultrasound scan was compared to the findings of the physical examination tests (Neer's sign, Hawkins and Kennedy test, painful arc of abduction, empty and full can tests, resisted isometric abduction and external rotation, which were regarded as either positive or negative. |
Data analysis		
Descriptive statistics were used to summarise prevalence.	Descriptive statistics were used to summarise the responses and the Chi-squared statistic was used if responses appeared to differ according to level of special-interest.	Sensitivity, specificity, likelihood ratios and overall accuracy were calculated for each physical examination test.
Findings		
Point prevalence of shoulder tendinitis was 88/2743 (3.2%).	The respondents would undertake a wide range of diagnostic tests, offer a wide variety of treatment and offer a broad prediction of prognosis.	These physical examination tests have limited capacity to inform diagnosis.

Table 7.1 Summary of included studies

CHAPTER EIGHT

RANDOMISED CONTROLLED TRIAL

Introduction

The randomised controlled trial is regarded by many as the most appropriate research design to evaluate the effectiveness of an intervention (Littlewood 2011). As described in chapter two, there are three key components to a randomised controlled trial. Firstly, the research participants are allocated to two or more groups *randomly*, meaning by chance. Secondly, in its most basic form, research participants are allocated to the intervention or *control* group. Thirdly, the intervention group is compared to the control group in order to evaluate whether one group has performed better than the other and hence whether one treatment is more effective than another (Torgerson and Torgerson 2008).

Despite being held in such high regard by many, it is not uncommon for apparently similar randomised controlled trials to present conflicting conclusions. This conflict might be explained by the quality of these different studies and their inherent risk of bias (van der Windt and Bouter 2003). Thus, to enable useful interpretation and application of research it is necessary to critically appraise studies to enable the validity of their results to be understood (Crombie 1996). Hence, the following section will offer a critical appraisal of three randomised controlled trials that aimed to evaluate the effectiveness of various interventions in the management of rotator cuff disorders. The studies are summarised in table 8.1.

Critical appraisal

The three studies to be appraised are: Bang and Deyle (2000), Brox et al (1993), Ludewig and Borstad (2003). There are numerous quality appraisal tools for analysing the methodological rigour of randomised controlled trials, more than for any other study design. However the different tools usually focus on much the same aspects of study methodology, which will provide the structure for this critique.

Research aims and research questions

All studies had clearly stated aims including comparisons of various exercise programmes, incorporating loaded exercise, with manual therapy (Bang and Deyle 2000), surgery (Brox et al 1993) and no intervention (Ludewig and Borstad 2003). This enables a clear judgement about the relevance of the studies to practice to be made, which is a strength of the research. Where a clear statement of aim is not made it has also been suggested that this is indicative of poor writing and usually poor quality research (Schulz et al 2010) which means that the results of the study should be treated with caution.

Research approach/design

All studies were randomised controlled trials which, when conducted to a high standard, are regarded as the gold standard for evaluating the effectiveness of an intervention (Higgins and Green 2008). Thus, the research designs were appropriate to answer the research questions. However, although the randomised controlled trial is an appropriate design, the manner in which the trials are conducted needs to be appraised before accepting the findings (Herbert et al 2005). It has been suggested that sub-optimal methods of allocation in randomised controlled trials may lead to an over-exaggeration of treatment effect (Higgins and Green 2008). Only Ludewig and Borstad (2003) reported their method of randomisation which includes measures to conceal the allocation from participants, therapists and researchers. Bang and Deyle (2000) did not mention their method of randomisation or any attempts to conceal allocation whereas Brox et al (1993) referred to allocation by the method of random permuted blocks, which is an accepted method (Bowling 2002), but did not mention any attempt to conceal allocation. Due to the influence that the method of allocation might have on reported treatment effect the results of Bang and Deyle (2000) and Brox et al (1993) should be treated with caution (Higgins and Green 2008). In presenting the updated guidelines for reporting parallel group randomised trials Moher et al (2010) provide further detail relating to the process of randomisation and the consequences of sub-optimal methods in addition to other important aspects of randomised controlled trials methodology.

Sampling

The sampling procedures of Bang and Deyle (2000) and Brox et al (1993) represented usual practice where participants were recruited post referral to the treatment centre. This adds credibility in the form of external validity or generalisability where the research methods are aligned to real world practice (Greenhalgh 2010). However, Ludewig and Borstad (2003) recruited local construction journeymen through local unions and safety meetings and hence should be regarded as a non-clinical population. So, even if this study is regarded as credible in terms of internal validity, i.e. the extent to which a research study is free of bias, the use of a non-clinical population limits the external validity of the findings, i.e. the extent to which findings from the research sample can be inferred to the wider population.

Brox et al (1993) and Ludewig and Borstad (2003) were the only studies to provide evidence of a sample size calculation. The failure to do this has both ethical and scientific implications. A sample size calculation is an accepted means of estimating the required number of participants needed to detect a true treatment effects between groups if one does actually exist (Dawson and Trapp 2001). Bang and Deyle (2000) did not justify their sample size but did identify a statistically significant difference between their groups which means that a Type II error did not occur in this situation (Bowling 2002). However, Bang and Deyle (2000) only recruited 52 participants in total which might be seen to compromise the external validity of the study due to the low numbers.

Data collection

All studies used different measures of outcome and followed up their participants at different times. This is a serious shortcoming in this body of literature which challenges the possibility of synthesising the results of the studies. Only one study (Ludewig and Borstad 2003) clearly stated that they used measures of outcome that had been validated in the population in which they were investigating. Validity relates to how truthful a measure is (Bowling 2001). If an outcome measure is selected which has not been validated in the chosen population it should be regarded as compromising the internal validity of the study and again the results of Bang and Deyle (2000) and Brox et al (1993) should be treated with caution.

In concluding that manual therapy was a useful additional intervention for participants with subacromial impingement syndrome, Bang and Deyle (2000) measured pain levels at three to four weeks and function at two months. This selective short term outcome measurement in favour of one of the treatment arms is a potential source of bias and hence the conclusions drawn might be challenged.

All studies have taken steps to minimise researcher bias when collecting the data from the outcome measures. Bang and Deyle (2000) and Brox et al (1993) incorporated assessor blinding while Ludewig and Borstad (2003) asked participants to independently complete the measures. Not forgetting the limitations of the measures used, methods to minimise assessor bias should be regarded as a strength as this minimises any biases that the assessor might have about the results.

Data analysis

All studies reported using statistical techniques which are accepted for determining between group differences (Field 2009). Appendix A of this book includes an algorithm to help readers determine whether an appropriate statistical test has been used when appraising other studies and chapter ten includes a description of the reasoning process relating to this algorithm; to minimise the potential for grey matter overload that process is not repeated here. Consideration of whether the results are statistically significant is presented in all papers but the issue of clinical significance warrants further thought; especially since some of the reported measures are not validated. As mentioned, Ludewig and Borstad (2003) used an outcome measure that has been validated, i.e. the Shoulder Rating Questionnaire, but a mean change of 9.9 points on this measure is not regarded as clinically significant (L'Insalata et al 1997). This is an important consideration because currently the clinicians might ask: *"What does this actually mean for my patients and me?"*

However, two recognised threats to internal validity include whether data analysis was undertaken on an intention-to-treat basis and whether missing data was dealt with appropriately (Higgins and Green 2008). Intention-to-treat analysis refers to whether the participant's data was analysed according to the group they were allocated to as opposed to the treatment that they actually received (Higgins and Green 2008). Brox et al (1993) reported using an intention-to-treat method but do not report how they dealt with missing values. The impact of this is unclear but might be significant considering that approximately 30% of participants in the surgery group were not followed up at three months and approximately 10% were lost to follow-up at six months. Ludewig and Borstad (2003) described analysing the data of all subjects for whom post-test data was obtained. This implies that some participants were lost to follow-up but the authors do not report this number or the reasons for drop-out which casts doubt upon the validity of the analysis. Bang and Deyle (2000) reported that they collected complete data sets from all but one of their subjects which suggests that bias, due to incomplete follow-up, is likely to be minimal but intention-to-treat analysis was not reported and it appears that no consideration was given to the fact that participants might receive other therapy, for example the exercise group receiving manual therapy, during the study period.

Findings

In the study by Bang and Deyle (2000) both groups experienced statistically significant reductions in pain and improvement in function but this was greater in the combined treatment group. With regards to pain, the change could also be regarded as clinically significant according to amount of change on the outcome measure used. In the study by Brox et al (1993) no statistically or clinically significant differences between the surgical and exercise group were detected but both improved significantly more than the placebo group. In the study by Ludewig and Borstad (2003) there were statistically significant changes in favour of the exercise group.

Generalisability

The relatively small sample sizes of the studies limits generalisability but Brox et al (1993) and Ludewig and Borstad (2003) did justify their sample sizes. All of the studies provide clear detail of the criteria that participants had to meet in order to enter the trial. This is important because it enables a judgement regarding applicability, i.e. are the participants in the study sufficiently similar to those seen in clinical practice? (Moher et al 2010). Bang and Deyle (2000) and Brox et al (1993) included participants recruited from a clinical environment which could enhance the transferability of their findings, but caution should be exercised when interpreting findings from Ludewig and Borstad (2003) where an all-male non-clinical population was recruited which might be significantly different from a clinical population due to possible confounding factors, for example motivation, psychological disposition, co-morbidity.

Implications and usefulness

In summary, the evidence presented suggests that exercise might be more beneficial than no intervention, at least as beneficial as surgery with additional benefit conferred when complemented by manual therapy. However, although the study by Ludewig and Borstad (2003) appeared to be of a higher methodological quality, all of the studies have a potentially high risk of bias and/or imprecision. So, the value of all of the reviewed studies in terms of influencing clinical decision making is limited. Despite the limitations of the studies, these findings offer a platform upon which to develop future ideas. There is a need for further randomised controlled trials which recruit a justified sample size from a specified clinical population. These trials need to utilise and report appropriate methods of random allocation, for example distance computer-generated random allocation, along with validated measures of outcome, for example the Shoulder Pain and Disability Index, with appropriate length of follow-up, for example three, six and 12 months, to capture meaningful data.

Summary

This chapter has recognised the strengths and limitations of some randomised controlled trials that have evaluated the effectiveness of various interventions in the treatment of rotator cuff disorders. The implications of these strengths and limitations have been discussed. The chapter has recognised the limitations of this research which suggests that high quality research needs to be undertaken to further inform clinical practice.

Reproduced from Manual Therapy, 16(6), Littlewood C, The RCT means nothing to me! 2011, p. 614-7. Copyright (2011), with permission from Elsevier.

References

Bang M and Deyle G (2000). Comparison of supervised exercise with and without manual physical therapy for patients with shoulder impingement syndrome. Journal of Orthopaedic and Sports Physical Therapy, 30(3), 126-37.

Bowling A (2001). Measuring disease (2nd edition). Open University Press, Buckingham.

—. (2002). Research methods in health care (2nd edition). Open University Press, Maidenhead.

Brox J, Staff P, Ljungren A, Brevik J (1993). Arthroscopic surgery compared with supervised exercises in patients with rotator cuff disease. British Medical Journal, 307, 899-903.

Crombie I (1996). Research in health care. John Wiley and Sons Ltd, Chichester, UK.

Dawson B and Trapp R (2001). Basic and clinical biostatistics (3rd edition). McGraw-Hill, London, UK.

Field A (2009). Discovering statistics using SPSS (3rd edition). Sage Publications, UK.

Greenhalgh T (2010). How to read a paper (4th edition). Wiley-Blackwell, Chichester,UK.

Herbert R, Jamtdedt G, Mead J, Birger Hagen K (2005). Practical evidence based physiotherapy. Elsevier Butterworth-Heinemann, Edinburgh, UK.

Higgins J and Green S (2008). Cochrane handbook of systematic reviews. Wiley-Blackwell, Chichester,UK.

L'Insalata J, Warren R, Cohen S, Altchek D, Peterson M (1997). A self-administered questionnaire for assessment of symptoms and function of the shoulder. Journal of Bone and Joint Surgery 79, 738-48.

Littlewood C (2011). The RCT means nothing to me! Manual therapy, 16, 614-617.

Ludewig P and Borstad J (2003). Effects of a home exercise programme on shoulder pain and functional status in construction workers. Occupational and Environmental Medicine, 60, 841-9.

Moher D, Hopewell S, Schulz K, Montori V, Gotzsche P, Devereaux P et al (2010). CONSORT 2010 explanation and elaboration: updated guidelines for reporting parallel group randomised trials. Journal of Clinical Epidemiology, 63, 1-37.

Schulz K, Altman D, Moher D (2010). CONSORT 2010 statement: updated guidelines for reporting parallel group randomised trials. British Medical Journal, 340, 698-702.

Torgerson D, Torgerson C (2008). Designing randomised trials in health, education and the social sciences. Palgrave Macmillan; Basingstoke.

Van der Windt D, Bouter L (2003). Physiotherapy or corticosteroid injection for shoulder pain? Annals of Rheumatic Diseases, 62(5), 385-7

Author/ date/ title	Bang and Deyle (2000). Comparison of supervised exercise with and without manual physical therapy for patients with shoulder impingement syndrome.	Brox et al (1993). Arthroscopic surgery compared with supervised exercises in patients with rotator cuff disease.	Ludewig and Borstad (2003). Effects of a home exercise programme on shoulder pain and functional status in construction workers.
Research question/ aim	To compare a supervised shoulder exercise programme with a supervised exercise programme combined with manual therapy in shoulder impingement syndrome.	To compare the effect of arthroscopic subacromial decompression, a supervised exercise regime and placebo laser treatment in patients with rotator cuff pathology.	To compare a therapeutic exercise programme with no treatment in patients with shoulder impingement syndrome.
Research design	Randomised controlled trial. Single blinding only – outcome assessor. Short-term follow-up of pain at 3-4 weeks and short-term follow-up of function at 2 months.	Randomised controlled trial. Single blinding only – outcome assessor. Mid-term follow-up at 6 months.	Randomised controlled trial. Short-term follow up only at 2-3 months.
Sample	52 patients referred by a physician with a diagnosis of impingement or rotator cuff tendinitis. 58% male, mean age 43 years. Inclusion criteria include positive impingement test and pain with active abduction or resisted test.	125 patients referred by their general medical practitioner with a diagnosis of rotator cuff disease. 53% male, mean age 48 years. Inclusion criteria include pain with shoulder abduction, largely maintained range of movement and pain with resisted tests.	67 volunteer construction workers were recruited through local unions and safety meetings. 100% male, mean age 49 years. Inclusion criteria include shoulder pain exacerbated with resisted testing and largely maintained range of movement.

Data Collection		
The visual analogue scale (VAS) was used as a measure of pain. Function was measured with an unvalidated assessment questionnaire developed by the authors from the Oswestry Disability Index.	The Neer shoulder score was used as the primary outcome measure.	The shoulder rating questionnaire and the shoulder pain and disability index, which have been validated for use in populations with shoulder pain, were the primary outcome measures.
Data analysis		
Multivariate analysis of variance was used to analyse between-group differences taking into account the interaction of the independent variables.	The Kruskal Wallis analysis of variance and Mann-Whitney U-test were used to assess within-group and between-group differences.	The analysis of variance was used to assess between-group differences.
Findings		
Both groups experienced statistically significant reductions in pain and improvement in function but this was greater in the combined treatment group. With regards to pain, the change could be regarded as clinically significant also.	No statistically or clinically significant differences were evident between the surgical and exercise group but both improved significantly more than the placebo laser group.	There were statistically significant changes in favour of the exercise group.

Table 8.1 Summary of included studies

CHAPTER NINE

NON-RANDOMISED TRIAL

Introduction

The non-randomised trial or quasi-experimental study, as it is frequently referred to, includes a control group and is a research design used to evaluate interventions but, unlike the randomised controlled trial, research participants are not allocated to the intervention or control group randomly. Other, non-random, means of allocation are used which might include the geographical region, the clinic visited or the physiotherapist seen.

Although there might be reasons for allocating participants in a non-random manner it should be recognised that this is still a source of selection bias, meaning that the study groups are potentially systematically different from one another at the outset of the study (Torgersen and Torgersen 2008). This systematic difference makes comparison difficult because if the groups are different to begin with then you can be reasonably sure that they will be different at the end of the study period, irrespective of what you do. It is common to observe that patients who report persistent pain and disability at the outset tend to still complain of persistent pain and disability at the end of a study compared to those who reported pain and disability of shorter duration initially, which highlights the point.

To explain the impact of selection bias let's consider an example. We are interested to know whether this book improves the knowledge of physiotherapists who are currently studying research methods. So, during the next seminar we take a number of copies of the book and distribute them to the half of the class who sit nearest to the front; clearly this is appropriate because it is most convenient. However, we also know that the most able students who consistently engage with the reading material sit nearest the front of the class as opposed to students who sit at the back of the class and snooze or engage with social media. We tell the students that we would like to assess their knowledge of research methods and to achieve this we will set a test in one week. The students then leave to prepare, the lucky front half with this book under their arm! One week later they return and complete the test which we mark eagerly and are relieved, and quite pleased, to see that the students who received this book performed significantly better on the test than the students who did not receive the book. Our conclusion; this book is brilliant and equips students with a thorough understanding of research methods. Correct? How can we be sure that the superior test results are due to engagement with the book and are simply not a product of the selection process where the more able and engaging students were allocated to receive the book? The answer is we can't and this is an example of the potential impact of selection bias. This means that results from non-randomised trials should always be treated with a degree of caution.

With these thoughts in mind, the following section will offer a critical appraisal of three non-randomised trials which focused on the impact of mass media campaigns on population back pain beliefs. The studies are summarised in table 9.1 and it is recommended that you review these summaries before reading the forthcoming sections of this chapter.

Critical appraisal

The three studies to be appraised are: Buchbinder et al (2001), Werner et al (2008) and Gross et al (2010).

Research question/ aim

All three studies provided clear aims describing an intention to evaluate the effectiveness of mass media campaigns on the beliefs that people hold about low back pain. Many health professionals think that if patients believe that rest is an appropriate way to manage an episode of low back pain then their recovery will be delayed. The media campaigns were designed to challenge this and other commonly-held negative beliefs which should, in theory, then improve the outcome from an episode of low back pain.

Research design

All three studies are non-randomised trials / quasi-experimental studies and describe using non-random methods to allocate participants to the intervention, i.e. mass media campaign, or control groups, i.e. no intervention in these cases. As mentioned above, the main concern here is selection bias where the intervention and control groups are imbalanced.

The authors of the studies report that the intervention and control groups were comparable in terms of the known factors that were measured including age and gender. However, it must be recognised that other, possibly unknown and immeasurable, factors might influence outcome. The process of random allocation to intervention and control groups in a randomised controlled trial results in comparable distribution of these known and unknown factors, known as confounding factors, which enables a fair comparison of outcome but this is compromised when non-random methods of allocation are employed.

Gross et al (2010) suggested that, because the campaign was delivered to the entire population, via radio, advertisements on buses and public service announcements, it was not possible to randomly allocate the participants to receive the intervention or control because everyone in the state (province) would be exposed due to the nature of the media chosen. It is simply not possible to tell some people to look at advertisements and others not. This is a similar issue for the other two studies and whereas this might be true when attempting to allocate individuals, it does not recognise the role of cluster randomised controlled trials. In a cluster randomised controlled trial the unit of allocation is a cluster, for example a geographical area, a hospital ward, a care home, rather than an individual (Torgersen and Torgersen 2008). Hence the clusters are randomly allocated as a means of minimising selection bias. So, why wasn't this undertaken in these studies? Closer inspection reveals that one of the studies (Buchbinder et al 2001) appears to have been exclusively funded by a body based in the state in which the media campaign was delivered and the researchers were required to evaluate the impact of this campaign. Hence, in tandem with the prohibitive expense of mass-media campaigns, it seems that conducting the intervention in the pre-selected, non-randomly allocated, state was the only option. In this situation pragmatism and reality overruled scientific ideal. The other studies describe a wider scope of funding beyond the state in which the media campaigns were delivered and it is unclear why random methods of allocation were not implemented at the cluster level.

Sample/ context

All of the studies reported administration of the mass media intervention to the entire population of the states/ provinces involved. For Buchbinder et al (2001), in Australia, the intervention state was Victoria and the control state was New South Wales. For Werner et al (2008), in Norway, Vestfold and Aust-Agder served as intervention counties and the control county was Telemark. For Gross et al (2010), in Canada, the intervention state was Alberta and Saskatchewan served as the control. Gross et al (2010) offer some justification as to why Alberta was selected as an intervention state because previous research had indicated that the population of this geographical location held pessimistic beliefs about low back pain. If it is accepted that addressing pessimistic beliefs is desirable, then from a public health perspective it can be seen why it would be appropriate to deliver an intervention in this context. However, from a research perspective this might give rise to some concern due to a concept known as regression to the mean which refers to movement towards the average score, in this case back beliefs, over time, irrespective of any intervention (Torgersen and Torgersen 2008). This is a phenomenon that some physiotherapists might be aware of in a clinical situation; when a patient with severe low back pain attends for treatment they will generally gradually improve with time even if the prescribed treatment is ineffective. In the case of Gross et al (2010) regression to the mean does not appear to have been a feature because the back belief scores remained fairly consistent over time in the intervention group but diminished slightly in the control group, indicating more pessimistic views. Despite this, the concept of regression to the mean should always be thought of, particularly when selection bias is a concern.

With regard to the other studies, Buchbinder et al (2001) evaluated the impact of the campaign in Victoria because the managers of the state's workers compensation system identified a need to address unhelpful beliefs in an attempt to reduce back pain compensation claims. The rationale for the selection of the states by Werner et al (2008) is unclear which limits the opportunity to fully appraise this aspect of the study.

Data collection

Both Buchbinder et al (2001) and Gross et al (2010) reported using computer-assisted telephone interviews to assess changes in beliefs according to the back beliefs questionnaire. Werner et al (2008) used a similar interview technique but changes in beliefs were based upon true/false responses to seven statements derived from Deyo's myths of low back pain. Whether the different representations of back pain beliefs influence the outcomes of the study is unclear but should be borne in mind. It is likely that different questionnaires will offer different evaluations of a domain, for example beliefs about back pain, which means that comparison between studies is compromised. The studies were fairly consistent in terms of when the interviews were undertaken; prior to the intervention and then post intervention which, in contrast to the previous point, does facilitate comparison of the findings of the studies.

A very important point to recognise here is that all of the studies refer to collecting data from random samples of the population. This does not mean that the studies are randomised controlled trials. Randomised, in the context of a randomised controlled trial, refers to how participants are allocated to the intervention or control group. In all of these studies this was done in a non-random way. However, to facilitate the process of data collection, the researchers randomly sampled participants from the intervention and control populations. Why would they do this? The populations of the states involved are huge and any attempt to collect data from each and every participant would take vast amounts of time and resources, which in this context renders it impossible. Instead the researchers take a smaller random sample that they anticipate represents the wider intervention or control populations and so can be generalised to these populations. This is a rational and sound scientific method of data collection providing that adequate numbers of participants are reached. Unfortunately in all three studies, the response rates to the telephone interviews was generally lower than what was regarded as necessary by the authors of the studies which casts doubt upon whether the responses gained are truly representative of the wider populations involved.

Data analysis

With these studies it is quite easy to get lost in the complexity of the analyses. Buchbinder et al (2001) described using a two-way independent group analysis of variance (ANOVA) to evaluate the effect of state (Victoria or New South Wales) and time on back beliefs. This simply indicates that the effect of two independent variables (state and time; two-way) was evaluated on different groups (intervention and control state; independent) (Field 2009). In contrast, despite stating similar aims and collecting similar data, Gross et al (2010) report using multivariate linear regression to evaluate the effect of state (province) and time on back beliefs. Why the difference? Well, this is to do with how the researchers treated their raw data. Whereas Buchbinder et al (2001) treated state and time (wave 1, 2 or 3) as categorical variables, which is a requirement for ANOVA, Gross et al (2010) treated the state (province) as a categorical variable but it appears that they analysed time as a continuous variable and hence used regression instead. To add to this potential for confusion, Werner et al (2008) report using analysis of covariance (ANCOVA) with an interaction variable of time and state to test the effect of the media campaign over time on back beliefs.

Where to from here? Just as there is frequently more than one treatment that could be appropriately offered to a patient, there is frequently more than one approach to data analysis. Reference to a dedicated statistics book, for example Field (2009), assists us to make a judgement that these statistical techniques are appropriate for the data collected and appropriate to enable the aims of the studies to be met. However, it is unclear why the data has been treated in different ways, for example coding time as a continuous variable in one study and a categorical variable in another. It is also unclear whether these different approaches to data analysis could result in different outcomes. Perhaps consideration of this is beyond the scope of this book, so for now we accept that the analysis undertaken is valid and appropriate even though questions remain.

Findings

Buchbinder et al (2001) reported significant benefits in terms of population beliefs about low back pain, whereas Werner et al (2008) and Gross et al (2010) reported smaller improvements and questioned the significance of any changes in terms of disability and/ or health care utilisation. The authors of the studies reporting smaller or insignificant effects reflected upon the scope of their media campaigns and the amount of funding available to support them. The resources available were much less than those available to Buchbinder et al (2001) who appeared to employ a wider ranging campaign supported by greater funds which might explain the different results.

Implications and usefulness

The evidence reviewed suggests that mass-media campaigns have the potential to influence back pain beliefs which in turn might influence levels of disability and health care use but this could be dependent upon the scope and scale of the campaign and modest attempts at media campaigning might result in outcomes that are not particularly meaningful. At the level of the individual physiotherapist, these findings might be of limited use; particularly considering the limited impact that two of the studies had and considering the amount of money required to fund such campaigns. Despite some pragmatic reasons for undertaking non-randomised studies, there does seem to be opportunity to expose mass media campaigns to more robust evaluation through cluster randomised controlled trials to evaluate whether the outcomes reported by some hold true when the risk of selection bias is minimised.

Summary

This chapter has introduced the non-randomised trial/ quasi experimental study. Three published trials have been described and critically appraised. The critical appraisal has recognised some of the limitations of this research design and hence has offered a basis upon which the novice researcher can approach and critically appraise other similar studies.

References

Buchbinder R, Jolley D, Wyatt M (2001). Effects of a media campaign on back pain beliefs and its potential influence on management of low back pain in general practice. Spine, 26(23), 2535/2542.

Field A (2009). Discovering statistics using SPSS (3rd edition). Sage Publications, UK.

Gross D, Russell A, Ferrari R, Battie M, Schopflocher D, Hu R, Waddell G, Buchbinder R (2010). Evaluation of a Canadian back pain mass media campaign. Spine, 35(8), 906-913.

Torgerson D and Torgerson C (2008). Designing randomised trials in health, education and the social sciences. Palgrave Macmillan; Basingstoke.

Werner E, Ihlebaek C, Laerum E, Wormgoor M, Indahl A (2008). Low back pain media campaign. Patient education and counselling, 71, 198-203.

Author/ date/ title		
Buchbinder et al (2001). Effects of a media campaign on back pain beliefs and its potential influence on management of low back pain in general practice.	Werner et al (2008). Low back pain media campaign.	Gross et al (2010). Evaluation of a Canadian back pain mass media campaign.
Research question/ aim		
To evaluate the effectiveness of a population-based media campaign designed to alter beliefs about back pain.	To evaluate the effectiveness of a media campaign on popular beliefs about low back pain.	To evaluate the impact of the Alberta back pain mass media campaign on beliefs of the general population.
Research design		
Non-randomised trial/ quasi-experimental study.	Non-randomised trial/ quasi-experimental study.	Non-randomised trial/ quasi-experimental study.
Sample		
The entire population of Victoria, Australia were exposed to the campaign with New South Wales serving as the control.	The populations of Vestfold and Aust-Agder, Norway, were exposed to the campaign with Telemark serving as the control.	The entire population of Alberta, Canada were exposed to the campaign with an unexposed neighbouring province, Saskatchewan, serving as the control.
Data Collection		
Computer-assisted telephone interviews were undertaken to assess change in beliefs according to the back beliefs questionnaire. Interviews were undertaken prior to the intervention and then two and 2 ½ years afterwards from a random sample of the population.	Computer-assisted telephone interviews were undertaken to assess change in beliefs based upon true/ false responses to seven statements derived from Deyo's myths of low back pain. Interviews were undertaken prior to the intervention, during the intervention and then at its conclusion from a random sample of the population.	Computer-assisted telephone interviews were undertaken to assess change in beliefs according to the back beliefs questionnaire. Interviews were undertaken prior to the intervention and then annually afterwards for three years from a random sample of the population.

Non-randomised Trial

Data analysis		
Two-way independent group analysis of variance (ANOVA) was used to evaluate the effect of state and time on back beliefs.	Analysis of covariance (ANCOVA) with an interaction variable of time x state to test the effect of the campaign over time on back beliefs.	Multivariate linear regression was used to evaluate the effect of province and time on back beliefs.
Findings		
There were statistically significant improvements ($p < 0.001$) over time in back belief questionnaire scores in Victoria but not New South Wales.	There were small but statistically significant ($p<0.001$) changes in beliefs about low back pain favouring the intervention states.	The interaction between province and time was not statistically significant ($p = 0.13$) which suggests no meaningful effect of the campaign on back belief questionnaire scores.

Table 9.1 Summary of included studies

Chapter Ten

Uncontrolled Trial

Introduction

The term uncontrolled trial refers to a trial without a control group; there is only one experimental group. Some texts will describe these studies as before and after studies because usually a measurement is taken before, and then after, an experimental intervention.

Having read chapter two about research design and chapter eight about the randomised controlled trial, where the importance of random allocation to groups alongside the need for a control group to adequately judge whether an intervention is effective was emphasised, might lead you to question the role and value of an uncontrolled study. This is an appropriate question to ponder and one that will be considered now. Evaluating the effectiveness of an intervention is not strictly the purpose of an uncontrolled study or trial, although often reported in the literature as such. Instead, an uncontrolled trial is most commonly used as a feasibility study. That is an assessment of how feasible it would be to undertake a randomised controlled trial which requires more time and is much more costly. A feasibility study typically involves a relatively small number of participants but enables an understanding of whether there are sufficient patient numbers to carry out a randomised controlled trial and also enables an estimate of how long it might take to recruit the required numbers. Also, a feasibility study enables the questionnaires or outcome measures to be used in practice to evaluate how acceptable they are to the patient group and how long they might take to complete; both important considerations when planning for a randomised controlled trial. Furthermore, it is possible that the intervention or treatment to be researched has not been widely used before and so it is necessary to examine the acceptability before it is rolled out in a wider setting. Imagine the implications of beginning a randomised controlled trial and seeing all the participants randomised to the intervention group dropping out because the intervention is not acceptable to them due to, for example, time constraints; this would be catastrophic and a huge waste of resources.

Despite this, there are times when an uncontrolled trial might be the best available option to evaluate the effectiveness of an intervention. Researchers might think it unethical to randomly allocate participants to intervention or control groups, for example when one treatment is regarded as being far superior to possible comparators or control treatments. In this situation equipoise, or ambivalence regarding the superiority of one treatment over the other, which is widely regarded as a necessary basis for randomisation, is compromised (Herbert et al 2005). The ramifications of this are that clinicians might be asked to deliver interventions that they do not believe are useful or effective which is clearly not a favourable, or ethical, situation. Also there might be insufficient number of participants to populate an intervention and control group. Even in circumstances where the uncontrolled trial might be regarded as the best available option, it should still be remembered that selection bias is probable and the lack of an appropriate control group against which a treatment can be adequately evaluated means that any attempts to evaluate the effectiveness of an intervention using an uncontrolled study design should be treated with extreme caution.

With these thoughts in mind, the following section will offer a critical appraisal of three uncontrolled trials which focused on specific exercise programmes for people with shoulder pain. The studies are summarised in table 10.1 and it is recommended that you review these summaries before reading the forthcoming sections of this chapter.

Critical appraisal

The three studies to be appraised are: Jonsson et al (2005), Camargo et al (2009) and Bernhardsson et al (2010).

Research question/ aim

All three studies provided clear aims describing an intention to evaluate the effectiveness of exercise-based treatment regimes in people with impingement syndrome, which is regarded as a common type of shoulder pain. Although clear aims are presented, as we have seen, these do not align with the purpose of an uncontrolled trial.

Research design

The reports from the studies refer to various designs including pilot study (Jonsson et al 2005), single-subject (Bernhardsson et al 2010) and clinical trial (Camargo et al 2009). Despite this variation in reporting, all of the studies should be regarded as uncontrolled trials because one sample of participants was recruited, baseline measures of pain and disability were taken, an intervention was offered as part of the research and then the measures were repeated.

When considered with reference to the reported aims of the studies, the uncontrolled trial design is not appropriate to enable a valid evaluation of the effectiveness of an intervention. Without a control group it is not possible to conclude that an intervention is effective or not, because change might be due to the passage of time rather than the intervention. Many musculoskeletal problems tend to vary in their presentation and people will tend to seek health care at the point of maximal need, i.e. when their pain or disability is at its worst. We know that many conditions improve with time, whether they receive treatment or not, a concept known as regression to the mean. So, any positive health gains in patients needs to be judged in the context of knowing that improvement would tend to take place anyway. A control group accounts for changes in pain and/or disability due to factors other than the treatment. This then means that any difference in health gain (or deterioration) *between* an intervention and control group can be attributed to the effects of the experimental treatment, providing that the groups were comparable to begin with! This was considered in more depth in chapter 0.

When these studies are considered in the wider context of the shoulder pain literature an argument for the suitability of the design can be made. Jonsson et al (2005) were investigating painful eccentric exercises for chronic painful impingement syndrome. Such an approach is not aligned with the way that most physiotherapists would treat people with this problem (Littlewood et al 2012) and so an uncontrolled trial has the potential benefit of ascertaining whether such an approach to treatment is acceptable to the treating therapists and also the patients. However, this information was not reported. Bernhardsson et al (2010) recognised the paucity of research in this field and hence the limited literature that was available to inform the development of a suitable exercise programme. Again, in this situation, a small scale uncontrolled trial is appropriate to assess the feasibility of the exercise programme, but factors including adherence to the programme and acceptability were not reported. Camargo et al (2009) recruited participants from an occupational setting as opposed to the more typical clinical setting. Such a difference in setting might have implications for the rate of recruitment to a randomised controlled trial and so it is appropriate to determine the feasibility of recruiting participants before undertaking the definitive randomised controlled trial.

It should be noted that all the reports do recognise the limitations of their study designs and all conclude with recognition that randomised controlled trials are needed to fully evaluate the effectiveness of the interventions. This highlights that the uncontrolled trial was appropriate to determine the feasibility of further studies but was not appropriate to evaluate the effectiveness of the interventions.

Sample/ context

The three studies take different approaches to recruitment. Jonsson et al (2005) recruited nine participants who had already received conservative treatment, including physiotherapy, and were on the waiting list for surgical treatment in Sweden. Camargo et al (2009) recruited a sample of 14 male participants from an occupational setting in Brazil. It appears that these participants were not currently receiving health care or had not received healthcare recently because participants were excluded from the study if they had received a corticosteroid injection within the last three months or physiotherapy within the last six months. Bernhardsson et al (2010) recruited ten participants from primary health care clinics in western Sweden.

The contrast between these studies is clear. Camargo et al (2009) recruited a sample of non-healthcare seeking participants who were presumably functioning at a reasonable level because they continued to work. A little further down the spectrum of severity, Bernhardsson et al (2010) recruited participants who were accessing primary healthcare services while Jonsson et al (2005), towards the end of the severity spectrum, recruited participants who had not responded to healthcare thus far and were awaiting surgical input. It is fair to expect that responses in terms of feasibility and treatment outcome would be different across these different samples and contexts and this should be considered when interpreting any results. For example, in many situations high levels of baseline pain and disability tend to predict a poor treatment outcome and it would be expected that those who have opted for surgical treatment would tend to be at the more severe end of the spectrum and be complaining of higher pain and disability compared to those who continue to work, i.e. Jonsson et al's sample compared to Camargo et al's sample.

These differences also have to be taken into account if readers are attempting to generalise the findings of these studies to their own practice, i.e. *do these participants represent the patients I encounter?* In addition to this consideration, extreme caution should be exercised if attempting to generalise the findings of these studies due to the small number of participants included.

Data collection

As with most trials, Jonsson et al (2005), Camargo et al (2009) and Bernhardsson et al (2010) used a range of outcome measures (questionnaires) to evaluate the effect of the treatments they were investigating. Among others, Jonsson et al (2005) and Bernhardsson et al (2010) utilised the Constant score which is a commonly used measure to evaluate shoulder function. The Constant score combines the patient's self-report of pain and activities of daily living with measures of range of movement and strength (Roy et al 2010). It is regarded as a valid measure, i.e. it measures what it intends to measure, namely shoulder function (Roy et al 2010). It is regarded as a reliable measure, i.e. if the patient's status does not change between the completion of the initial measure and the next, then the Constant score achieved will be similar (Roy et al 2010). It is also regarded as a responsive measure, i.e. if the patient's status changes then this should be reflected by a change in the Constant score. So, in terms of critical appraisal, Jonsson et al (2005) and Bernhardsson et al (2010) have selected valid, reliable and responsive measures of outcome which should be regarded as a strength of these studies. Camargo et al (2009) utilised the Disabilities of the Arm, Shoulder and Hand (DASH) questionnaire to evaluate the treatment they were investigating. The DASH is also regarded as being valid, reliable and responsive and therefore should be considered an appropriate measure of outcome in this context (Roy et al 2009).

Most readers probably assume that appropriate outcome measures are always selected for research studies. Unfortunately, this is not the case and a brief review of the paper describing the study or a brief literature search should inform a critical appraisal before the measures are accepted as being appropriate.

Data analysis

In studies where quantitative data, i.e. numbers, are analysed, a number of decisions need to be taken before we know if the statistical test used is appropriate. To begin with, the level of data needs to be determined, i.e. is it nominal, ordinal, interval or ratio? (See the Glossary for an explanation of these terms) Nominal or ordinal data indicate the need for a non-parametric test whereas interval or ratio level data indicate that a parametric test might be appropriate.

With regards to the included studies, we are dealing with ordinal data, i.e. data that can be allocated to categories and can be ordered (Harris and Taylor 2004). Most self-report outcome measures used within physiotherapy research would be regarded as ordinal. To highlight this, consider the first item of the DASH which asks respondents to rate their ability to open a tight or new jar (www.dash.iwh.on.ca). The possible responses are

1) No difficulty
2) Mild difficulty
3) Moderate difficulty
4) Severe difficulty
5) Unable

Here the responses have been categorised and it is expected that someone rating their ability as having moderate difficulty would struggle to open the jar more than someone who rates their ability as mild or no difficulty. So, there is an order to the categories. You might be thinking, *"why isn't this data regarded as interval level data then?"* For data to be regarded as interval it must also be capable of being allocated to categories and be ordered, but the distance between the data points should be equal. So, moving from no difficulty to mild difficulty should represent the same change as moving from severe difficulty to unable or moderate difficulty to severe difficulty. Although these changes in status are represented by one point on the scale, can we be confident that a change in one point at any point on the scale is the same? It is generally accepted that we can't, so most scales of this nature are regarded as ordinal level and non-parametric tests are generally regarded as being the most appropriate. There are exceptions to this reasoning and this is an on-going debate within the wider statistical literature (Walters 2009), where, for now, it will stay!

Once we have decided that a non-parametric test is appropriate, we need to consider if we want to evaluate whether there is a difference or an association between our collected data. In the trials described here, the primary stated aims were to evaluate whether the participants reported an improvement from when they started treatment to when they finished. So, in this situation we are interested in determining a difference between two time points within the same group. Within-group differences are sometimes referred to as related or repeated measures. This is in contrast to between-group differences where the difference between two independent groups is to be evaluated. Think about within-group and between-group differences with reference to the uncontrolled trial, i.e. one group, and the randomised controlled trial, i.e. at least two groups, respectively. With this information we can now determine whether the tests used within the research study are appropriate. From table 10.1, it can be seen that all three trials used the Wilcoxon signed rank test, which, with reference to a statistical text book, e.g. Harris and Taylor (2004), we can determine is a non-parametric test for comparing the difference before and after treatment. Hence, based upon our reasoning, we can conclude that appropriate statistical analysis was undertaken.

Using the above reasoning process, Appendix A of this book includes an algorithm to help readers determine whether an appropriate statistical test has been used when appraising other studies.

Findings

Notwithstanding the previous comments regarding the appropriateness of the uncontrolled research design for evaluating the effectiveness of a treatment, the main results reported from the studies are summarised in table 10.1. Despite the different contexts in which the studies were undertaken and the different treatment regimens used, all of the studies reported statistically significant differences, i.e. there is less than 0.05 or 1/20 chance that these results would be observed if, in reality, there was no actual difference (if the null hypothesis (see glossary) were true) (Walters 2009). To explain this a little further, remember that there is always uncertainty with research and a chance that the results are wrong and this is why we refer to probability.

Camargo et al (2009) report a change which is also regarded as clinically significant, i.e. a change that would be recognised and valued by the patients and clinicians. The change of 12.67 points on the DASH exceeds what is regarded as the minimal clinical important difference of 10.2 (Roy et al 2009). However, alongside the mean estimate of 12.67 points is a range of values, 2.54 to 22.81, which represent the 95% confidence interval. This interval or range of values indicates where the true population value would lie (Walters 2009). To understand this point, again you need to recognise that research does not provide us with definitive answers in which we are 100% confident. There is always an element of uncertainty when trying to generalise the findings from a relatively small sample to the wider population and the smaller the sample the greater the uncertainty. The 95% confidence interval reflects this uncertainty and provides us with a range of values within which we are

95% confident that the true population value lies. So, in terms of the 95% confidence interval presented here, we are 95% confident that the true wider population value lies between 2.54 and 22.81. Hence it is possible that the intervention offered by Camargo et al (2009) would not be clinically significant in the wider population.

In relation to Jonsson et al (2005) and Bernhardsson (2010) who used the Constant score, although the change in score of 15.6 and 25 points appears impressive it is unclear whether these values are clinically significant. The reason for this is that the minimal clinical important difference for the Constant score has not been reported (Roy et al 2010). Whether the minimal clinical important difference has been established and reported is an important consideration when selecting an outcome measure so that the clinical value of the research outcome can be understood fully.

Even though we have mentioned that Jonsson et al (2005) report statistically significant findings it is interesting to note that, in doing this, these authors selected the data only from those participants who regarded themselves as being satisfied with treatment. A supplementary statistical analysis undertaken by us reveals that in those participants who indicated they were not satisfied, the mean change in Constant score was only 5.5 points and this was not statistically significant (p=0.273). When all participants were analysed together the mean change in Constant score was 11.2 points which again was not regarded as statistically significant (p=0.15). It is unclear why this analysis was omitted by Jonsson et al (2005) but fortunately the raw data was presented by the authors to enable further analysis to be undertaken which paints a different picture in relation to the primary outcome. It is possible that the lack of a statistically significant difference might reflect the small numbers of participants, which is another reason why such small uncontrolled trials should not aim to evaluate the effectiveness of treatments; but this lack of difference could also indicate that, on average, no effect can be attributed to the intervention.

Implications and usefulness

Due to the size of these trials in terms of numbers of participants and design in terms of the absence of a control group, little can be taken from these studies to help determine the effectiveness of the various exercise regimes. As the authors of these studies comment, these trials present a platform upon which further research of adequate size and design could be based but, from a clinical perspective, the implications are minimal. It seems that the usefulness of the studies could have been improved if the reporting had considered issues of feasibility which the authors and others could have considered when designing future research.

Summary

This chapter has introduced the uncontrolled trial. Three published trials have been described and critically appraised. The critical appraisal has recognised the role and limitations of the uncontrolled trial and has considered the implications of appropriate design including the sample and context of the study, the outcome measures used, the type of statistical analysis undertaken and the meaning of the results gained from such studies in relation to clinical practice and future research. The chapter has offered a basis upon which the novice researcher can approach and critically appraise other uncontrolled trial designs and/or begin to develop their own study.

References

Bernhardsson S, Klintberg I, Wendt G (2010). Evaluation of an exercise concept focusing on eccentric strength training of the rotator cuff for patients with subacromial impingement syndrome. Clinical Rehabilitation, 25(1), 69-78.

Camargo P, Haik M, Ludewig P, Filho R, Mattiello-Rosa S, Salvini T (2009). Effects of strengthening and stretching exercises applied during working hours on pain and physical impairment in workers with subacromial impingement syndrome. Physiotherapy Theory and Practice, 25(7), 463-475.

Harris M and Taylor G (2004). Medical Statistics Made Easy. Thomson Publishing Services, UK.

Herbert R, Jamtvedt G, Mead J, Hagen K (2005). Practical Evidence-Based Physiotherapy. Elsevier, UK.

Jonsson P, Wahlstrom P, Ohberg L, Alfredson H (2005). Eccentric training in chronic painful impingement syndrome of the shoulder: results of a pilot study. Knee Surgery, Sports Traumatology, Arthroscopy, 14(1), 76-81.

Littlewood C, Lowe A, Moore J (2012). Rotator cuff disorders: a survey of current UK physiotherapy practice. Shoulder and Elbow, 4(1), 64-71.

Roy J, MacDermid J, Woodhouse L (2009). Measuring shoulder function: a systematic review. Arthritis and Rheumatism, 61(5), 623-632.

Roy J, MacDermid J, Woodhouse L (2010). A systematic review of the psychometric properties of the Constant-Murley score. Journal of Shoulder and Elbow Surgery, 19, 157-164.

Walters S (2009). Quality of life outcomes in clinical trials and health-care evaluations. Wiley, UK.

Author/ date/ title		
Jonsson et al (2005). Eccentric training in chronic painful impingement syndrome of the shoulder: results of a pilot study.	Camargo et al (2009). Effects of strengthening and stretching exercises applied during working hours on pain and physical impairment in workers with subacromial impingement syndrome.	Bernhardsson et al (2010). Evaluation of an exercise concept focusing on eccentric strength training of the rotator cuff for patients with subacromial impingement syndrome.
Research question/ aim		
To investigate if treatment with painful eccentric muscle training was effective in patients with long-standing subacromial impingement syndrome.	To investigate if treatment with cryotherapy, strengthening and stretching exercises could be effective in workers with subacromial impingement syndrome.	To evaluate the effect of an eccentric strength training programme in patients with subacromial impingement syndrome.
Research design		
Uncontrolled trial	Uncontrolled trial	Uncontrolled trial
Sample		
Nine patients (5 male, 4 females) diagnosed with chronic painful impingement syndrome of the shoulder. Mean age 54 years (range 35 to 72). All patients had not responded to previous conservative treatments and were awaiting surgical intervention	Fourteen male assembly line workers diagnosed with subacromial impingement syndrome of the shoulder. Mean age 31 years.	Ten patients diagnosed with subacromial impingement of the shoulder. Mean age 54 years.

Data Collection		
The Constant score was used to assess shoulder function after 12 and 52 weeks of training.	The Disabilities of the Arm, Shoulder and Hand (DASH) questionnaire was used to assess shoulder function after 8 weeks of rehabilitation.	The Constant score was used to assess shoulder function after 12 weeks of training.
Patient satisfaction was assessed as 'yes or no' and those indicating 'yes' withdrew from the surgical waiting list.		
Data analysis		
Difference between before and after Constant score was evaluated with the Wilcoxon Signed Rank test.	Difference between before and after DASH score was evaluated with the Wilcoxon Signed Rank test.	Difference between before and after Constant score was evaluated with the Wilcoxon Signed Rank test.
Findings		
After 12 weeks of eccentric training, in those participants who indicated they were satisfied; mean change in Constant was score 15.6 points (p<0.043).	After 8 weeks of rehabilitation, the mean change in DASH score was 12.67 (95% CI 2.54 to 22.81) (p<0.05).	After 12 weeks of training, mean change in Constant score was 25 points (p = 0.008).

Table 10.1 Summary of included studies

CHAPTER ELEVEN

SYSTEMATIC REVIEW

Introduction

Systematic reviews, sometimes incorporating meta-analyses, tend to be placed at the top of the hierarchy of evidence, which we cautioned against uncritical acceptance of in chapter one. However, it is true to say that these studies are a vital source of evidence for busy working physiotherapists in a world in which hundreds of potentially relevant articles are appearing every month. Like all studies, systematic reviews should be conducted in a rigorous and reproducible manner, and thus represent good science, and take the quality of the included studies into account (Moher et al 2009). These are different from narrative reviews, which once were commonly seen in the medical and physiotherapy literature, but are less common these days. Greenhalgh (2010) suggests the following advantages of systematic reviews:

1) Explicit methods of data collection limit bias that, therefore, result in more reliable and accurate conclusions than old style narrative reviews
2) Large amounts of information can be assimilated quickly
3) Comparison between studies can establish if there is generalisability and consistency
4) Reasons for heterogeneity (differences), such as sub-groups, might be identified
5) Meta-analysis might increase the precision of the overall result.

Systematic reviews are sometimes termed secondary research, as they combine the results from multiple primary research papers. The essential features of a systematic review are a clearly defined and systematic search of the literature, explicit criteria to appraise the quality of the papers reviewed, and findings are analysed and synthesised in a meaningful and validated way (Gray 1997). A meta-analysis refers to a quantitative synthesis used as part of a systematic review. So, synthesis could be qualitative or narrative in nature, for example using a levels of evidence approach (see Littlewood et al 2012) or quantitative in nature where a single summary statistic is calculated (see Hayden et al 2005). Caution should be exercised when undertaking or interpreting a meta-analysis however because there should be an acceptable amount of homogeneity (similarity) across patient groups, interventions and outcomes, and the authors of the meta-analysis should demonstrate this. If due to heterogeneity of these study details a meta-analysis is not justified, a qualitative synthesis is more acceptable (Khan et al 2003). An inappropriate application of meta-analysis might occur if the results of studies evaluating the effect of exercise on low back pain are summed together as one. As physiotherapists we recognise that different exercises have different effects and we also recognise that different presentations of low back pain might respond differently to different exercise treatments. So, if different exercise programmes have different effects why would we want to sum them all together as one? Why would we then want to dilute this further by trying to summarise the effects of different exercise programmes on different presentations of low back pain, many of which might respond differently to the different programmes? We expect that most of you might suggest that this is not appropriate and so we caution against simplistic approaches to meta-analysis that do not adequately consider heterogeneity and recognise the clinical application of treatments when making decisions.

The advantage of systematic reviews should be clear from the outset; someone else has done the work of searching for, appraising, and synthesising the data on a particular topic. Systematic reviews should undoubtedly be the first choice if searching for answers on a specific topic. However systematic reviews do vary in quality, and as with primary studies, each must be appraised to determine the quality of its methods and findings and hence whether the findings should be accepted and then, if appropriate, applied to clinical practice.

Due to the recent explosion of the number of systematic reviews in the published literature, consideration has been given to critical appraisal of these types of studies rather than blind acceptance. Among others, is AMSTAR, a measurement tool to assess the methodological quality of systematic reviews (Shea et al 2007). This tool asks the following questions:

1) Was an 'a priori' design developed?
2) Was there duplicate study selection and data extraction?
3) Was a comprehensive literature search performed?
4) Was the status of publication used as an inclusion criterion?

5) Was a list of studies (included and excluded) provided?
6) Were the characteristics of the included studies provided?
7) Was the scientific quality of the included studies assessed and documented?
8) Was the scientific quality of the included studies used appropriately in formulating conclusions?
9) Were the methods used to combine the findings of the studies appropriate?
10) Was the likelihood of publication bias assessed?
11) Was any conflict of interest stated?

As with critical appraisal of primary studies, this process in relation to systematic reviews remains a work in progress and it remains unclear whether all of these criteria significantly impact upon the findings of a systematic review. However, it seems appropriate to at least consider these when evaluating a systematic review. With these thoughts in mind, the following section will offer a critical appraisal of three systematic reviews that have been selected, in part, to demonstrate the range of topics that can be evaluated with this methodology. The studies are summarised in table 11.1 and it is recommended that you review these summaries before reading the forthcoming sections of this chapter.

Critical appraisal

The systematic reviews to be appraised are May and Johnson (2008) which evaluates the effectiveness of stabilisation exercise for low back pain, McLean et al (2010) which investigates risk factors for non-specific neck pain and May et al (2010) which evaluates the reliability of physical examination tests used in the assessment of patients with shoulder pain.

Research aim and study design

All reviews clearly identified their aim in the title, but also justify the need for the review within the introduction. Justification of the need for a further review is important to minimise duplication and although previous reviews of stabilisation exercises had been published, May and Johnson (2008) identified more relevant published articles that had not been included in previous reviews and hence felt that further work was justified. With regard to McLean et al (2010) and May et al (2010), previous similar systematic reviews had not been undertaken and hence there was a clear indication to synthesise the primary data available.

Included studies

The focus of each of the reviews appraised here was different so clearly it was appropriate to include different study designs in each situation. May and Johnson (2008) were interested in the effectiveness of lumbar stabilisation exercise as an intervention so it was appropriate that only randomised controlled trials were included. For a review of risk factors for neck pain the included studies had to identify a pain-free population at baseline, with at least one-year follow-up and neck pain as the outcome of interest (McLean et al 2010). For the review of reliability of physical examination tests studies had to be reliability studies on patients with shoulder pain; asymptomatic individuals could only be included if the study involved patients with shoulder pain as well (May et al 2010). The included studies for all reviews appear to address the topic of the review. All reviews though excluded non-English papers, which could be seen as a potential source of language bias attributable to the lack of a truly comprehensive search strategy.

Data collection

All systematic reviews provided the search terms used in the search; they all used multiple electronic databases, and conducted hand searches of the reference lists of the articles obtained from the electronic search. These processes could have been enhanced by searching for unpublished literature and also by contacting experts in the field. Failure to do this raises questions about the comprehensiveness of the literature search and relevant papers might have been missed suggesting that publication bias might be a concern in these reviews.

In an attempt to minimise bias in the selection and data extraction processes, the included systematic reviews attempted to involve at least two reviewers during the study selection process and/or the data extraction process. This is important if you are contemplating conducting a systematic review, as misunderstandings or misinterpretations during the data-extraction process do occur. Some systematic reviews make comment on the level of agreement between reviewers when extracting data or making judgement about the quality of included studies. May et al (2010) reported kappa (a statistic for evaluating chance corrected agreement) values for agreement between those extracting the data as between 0.79 and 0.86 (May et al 2010), whereas McLean et al (2010) reported kappa values of 0.61. This indicates reasonable levels of agreement, but also provides evidence for the transparent nature of the data collection process and hence enhances validity or trustworthiness. This was not reported in the third systematic review.

Data analysis

All studies reported the method for evaluating the quality of the studies derived from previously used and published criteria. Outcomes were evaluated in different ways given the nature of the different study designs being reviewed, but all studies used strength or levels of evidence summaries as follows:

1) Strong = consistent findings from two or more high-quality studies
2) Moderate = consistent findings from at least one high quality study and one or more low-quality studies
3) Limited = findings from one high quality or one or more low quality studies
4) Conflicting = inconsistent findings irrespective of study quality.

May and Johnson (2008) reported Physiotherapy Evidence database (PEDro) scores for quality and p-values for differences between stabilisation exercises and the control group according to the duration of back pain, and the short, medium, or long-term outcome. May et al (2010) reported a previously used quality method for evaluating reliability studies, and used a pre-determined level of acceptable reliability, set at Kappa = 0.80, but as such cut-off points have an arbitrariness about them also conducted a sensitivity analysis at 0.70. McLean et al (2010) also used a set of criteria for judging quality that had been used in previous reviews for whiplash and non-specific neck pain, but adapted one item concerning sample size of the cohort studies to reflect the fact that there is less certainty regarding results in studies with smaller sample sizes. The interpretation of the results from the studies was clearly defined in the methods with the interpretation of p-values, and risk values being given a priori (before). In keeping with AMSTAR, it is important to state research methods prior to commencing a study to minimise the potential for bias. If researchers are allowed to change their methods without good reason as they go along, for example amending an exclusion criterion to omit a study that does not align with their own thinking, then bias will be introduced. As shown in these reviews, for all types of study design there are quality criteria available in the research literature, so the need for review authors to create their own set of quality criteria is highly unlikely.

Findings

The conclusions from all the reviews were reasonably definite, and unlikely to be changed by one or two papers that might have been missed. There was little evidence for the use of stabilisation exercise for acute low back pain; there was some evidence to support the use of stabilisation exercises for chronic low back pain. However the evidence was conflicting, and significant differences were less likely when compared to other active treatments, rather than inactive control groups, and, as treatments were mostly combined, the specific effect of stabilisation exercises was difficult to assess (May and Johnson 2008).

In the review of reliability studies for shoulder examination tests 36 studies were included; 17 of which were deemed to be of high quality. The majority of studies indicated poor reliability for all procedures investigated, with the high quality studies less likely to meet the pre-agreed acceptable level of reliability (May et al 2010). In the review of risk factors for neck pain 14 cohort studies were included, with all but one deemed to be of high quality (McLean et al 2010). There was strong evidence that high job demands, female gender, low social support, being an ex-smoker, and a history of previous neck or back pain was associated with future onset of neck symptoms.

Implications and usefulness

The widespread popularity of stabilisation exercises is not supported by the review of May and Johnson (2008). There is lack of evidence for their use in acute low back pain. There may be some evidence for their use in chronic low back pain but this is conflicting and appears to be no better than many other active exercise-based approaches. The review of May et al (2010) exposed the fact that there was little agreement between clinicians when they performed physical examination tests on patients with shoulder pain. Prior to this there had been numerous systematic reviews of physical examination procedures used in patients with shoulder pain that had challenged their validity, which is their ability to actually make the diagnosis that the test purported to do in comparison with a gold standard, such as findings at surgery. Hence, the fallacy of trying to make specific diagnoses from the clinical examination has been doubly exposed. Finally the review of McLean et al (2010) revealed groups who were more likely to develop neck pain in the future, for whom preventative strategies may be relevant and also demonstrated that demographic, psychosocial, and clinical factors were all relevant.

Summary

This chapter has introduced readers to the value of systematic reviews as summaries of evidence that have been collected with rigorous and reproducible methods, and provides a concise synthesis on a particular topic. As has been seen, this can relate to numerous subjects for which the way quality is assessed and the way the evidence might be summarised might vary; but the basic methodology remains the same. We have also offered a critical appraisal of three systematic reviews to allow readers to make judgements about systematic reviews that they might read, and also provide insight into how these reviews should be conducted.

References

Gray J (1997). Evidence-based Healthcare. How to Make Health Policy and Management Decisions Churchill Livingstone , New York.

Greenhalgh T (2010). How to read a paper (4th edition). Wiley-Blackwell, Chichester,UK.

Hayden J, van TulderM, Malmivaara A, Koes B (2005). Exercise therapy for treatment of non-specific low back pain. Cochrane Database of Systematic Reviews, 3.

Khan K, Kunz R, Kleijnen J, Antes G (2003). Systematic Reviews to Support Evidence-Based Medicine. How to review and Apply Findings of Healthcare research. The Royal Society Of Medicine Press Limited, London.

Littlewood C, Chance-Larsen K, May S, Sturrock B (2012). Exercise for rotator cuff tendinopathy: A systematic review. Physiotherapy, 98(2), 101-109.

May S and Johnson R (2008). Stabilisation exercises for low back pain: a systematic review. Physiotherapy, 94, 179-189.

May S, Chance-Larsen K, Littlewood C, Lomas D, Saad M (2010). Reliability of physical examination tests used in the assessment of patients with should pain: a systematic review. Physiotherapy, 96, 179-190.

McLean S, May S, Klaber-Moffett J, Sharp D, Gardiner E (2010). Risk factors for the onset of non-specific neck pain: a systematic review. Journal of Epidemiology and Community Health, 64, 565-572.

Moher D, Liberati A, Tetzlaff J, Altman DG et al (2009). Preferred reporting items for systematic reviews and meta-analyses: the PRISMA statement. British Medical Journal, 339, 332-336.

Shea B, Grimshaw J, Wells G, Boers M, Andersson N, Hamel C et al (2007). Development of AMSTAR: a measurement tool to assess the methodological quality of systematic reviews. BMC Medical Research Methodology, 7.

Reference / title /date	May and Johnson (2008). Stabilisation exercises for low back pain: a systematic review.	McLean et al (2010). Risk factors for the onset of non-specific neck pain: a systematic review.	May et al (2010). Reliability of physical examination tests used in the assessment of patients with should pain: a systematic review.
Research question / aim	As stated in title	As stated in title	As stated in title
Research design			
Systematic review	Systematic review	Systematic review	Systematic review
Included studies	Randomised controlled trials of adults with low back pain, one group treated with stabilisation exercises, outcomes of pain or disability (N = 18).	Prospective studies that recruited pain-free population at baseline, measured neck pain status at follow-up of at least 1 year (N = 14).	Reliability studies that included any patients with musculoskeletal shoulder pain or a mix of patients and asymptomatic volunteers and investigated physical examination procedures (N = 36).
Data collection	Medline, Cinahl, Amed, PEDro and the Cochrane database searched to October 2006; PEDro quality criteria were used to assess quality. Two reviewers independently extracted the data.	Medline, Cinahl, Amed, PEDro, Embase, PsychInfo and the Cochrane database searched to August 2007; a previously established set of 17 criteria was used to assess quality. Two reviewers independently extracted data.	Medline, PEDro, Amed, PsychInfo, Cinahl and the Cochrane database searched to June 2009; a previously used set of 14 criteria was used to assess quality. Two pairs of reviewers independently extracted data with a third if lack of consensus.
Data analysis	Due to heterogeneity of treatments, outcomes and population, a narrative synthesis was undertaken.	Due to heterogeneity of follow-up periods, outcomes, baseline variables, and data analysis, a narrative synthesis was undertaken.	Due to heterogeneity of tests, patients and analyses, a narrative synthesis was undertaken.

Findings
Little evidence to support stabilisation exercises for acute back pain. Some evidence in chronic back pain, but evidence was contradictory, and significant differences were less likely against active compared to inactive controls.
Female gender, older age, high job demands, low social support, being an ex-smoker, with a history of previous back or neck symptoms were linked to the development of neck pain.
No consistent evidence for any physical examination procedure to have acceptable reliability.

Table 11.1 Summary of included studies

Chapter Twelve

Challenges and Future Directions

We began this book by revisiting the meaning of evidence-based physiotherapy before considering the steps required to implement such a paradigm. From the outset, using the example of therapeutic ultrasound, it was clear that evidence-based physiotherapy is not an uncomplicated linear process. We have seen how research evidence indicates the potential benefit of one approach but real-world practice adopts or maintains another.

The reasons for such a mismatch of research evidence and clinical practice are multiple and include issues relating to the individual patient, the physiotherapist and the evidence base at our disposal. However, opportunities to implement evidence-based physiotherapy are there but are being missed or neglected. In our opinion, the current time lag to implementation of research evidence or the sheer denial of the existence of valid and applicable research evidence is not acceptable.

This book has attempted to stimulate critical thinking in the mind of the reader while encouraging them to access and appraise the wide range of research that is currently available. The time has come to question what we were taught and challenge the doctrines of gurus and opinion leaders. Within the paradigm of evidence-based physiotherapy it is no longer acceptable to do what we've always done. Within a framework of finite resources, new and emerging concepts will only thrive if old and redundant interventions and ways of clinical thinking are left behind.

The research evidence underpinning physiotherapy continues to evolve. We have seen throughout the chapters of this book that there are clear limitations to much of this evidence base, both in terms of validity or trustworthiness and applicability. However, there are clear messages emerging that we believe we can trust and apply to clinical practice.

More needs to be done to engage clinicians with research, both in terms of consumption and conduct. Platforms to begin to understand some of the complexity of the role of research within an evidence-based physiotherapy paradigm have been introduced but undoubtedly such a journey to enlightenment will be a marathon, not a sprint, and hopefully this book is a much needed water station in that marathon. On-going integration of research within the context of the evidence-based physiotherapy paradigm is needed, starting from pre-registration physiotherapy curricula, to post-registration curricula, and beyond into the world of real-world clinical practice.

It is unrealistic to expect that the future will bring the type and quality of research evidence that will enable us to make a decision about every individual patient that enters our clinic. Currently most research concerns groups of patients, for example groups of patients within randomised controlled trials, and average responses, for example mean reduction in pain, which can make implementation uncertain because we do not know how individual patients have responded within those groups. So, a mean group reduction in pain is a useful thing to know but within that group it is likely that some patients improved, some remained the same and some worsened but on average the response favours improvement. Hopefully you can see from this that a mean group improvement does not automatically infer that all individuals will improve. However, it is with knowledge of this uncertainty in tandem with an understanding of the expectations of our patients and our own clinical experience and expertise, that we can make optimal evidence-informed decisions in partnership with our patients.

It is within this perspective that recent randomised controlled trials have started to explore how sub-groups of patients respond to different interventions with, for instance, back pain or shoulder pain (Fritz et al 2003, Littlewood et al 2012). Traditional randomised controlled trials ignored possible heterogeneity within these groups and simply randomised patients to treatments regardless of whether or not they might be relevant to that patient. Treatments based on classification sub-groups might well be a way to make the results of randomised controlled trials more clinically relevant to individual patients and so to clinical practice.

Another key area in which traditional clinical thinking may need to be re-evaluated is regarding diagnosis based on specific structural pathology. This concept has been largely marginalised in the management of patients with low back pain, but its relevance to patients with non-spinal problems is being increasingly recognised. Studies into the validity and reliability of the assessment and classification process consistently challenge traditional assumptions that accurate diagnoses can definitely be made. Again this supports the value of a classification process using clinically-based classification sub-groups.

The future of a critically thinking profession is undoubtedly bright. The opportunity to improve physiotherapy at the "coalface" for the good of our patients is indeed an exciting but challenging one which requires a questioning approach to clinical practice, judicious consumption of research evidence and a tenacious attitude to implementation. In closing, if this book stimulates the reader to ask, *"Why do we do that? What does the research tell us? Can we trust the research evidence? Can we apply the research evidence to our practice?"* then we will have achieved our aim.

References

Fritz J, Delitto A, Erhard R (2003). Comparison of classification-based physical therapy with therapy based on clinical practice guidelines for patients with acute low back pain: a randomized clinical trial. Spine, 28, 1363-1372.

Littlewood C, Ashton J, Mawson S, May S, Walters S (2012). A mixed methods study to evaluate the clinical and cost-effectiveness of a self-managed exercise programme versus usual physiotherapy for chronic rotator cuff disorders: protocol for the SELF study. BMC Musculoskeletal Disorders, 13, 62.

GLOSSARY OF TERMS

Allocation concealment
A process where those who assign participants to a study are unaware of the sequence of future assignments.
Alternative hypothesis
The research statement you are looking to prove, for example, there is a difference between treatments.
Blinding
A process where patients, clinicians and outcome assessors are unaware of whether the patient has received the intervention or control treatment.
Case-control study
An observational study that recruits a group of people with a condition of interest or diagnosis (case), and a group of people similar to those with the condition or diagnosis but without the specific condition (controls) to investigate factors that might contribute to or protect from the development of a disease or condition.
Case series
A collection of multiple case studies.
Case study
A report or a description of some or all aspects of a patient encounter.
Categorical data (see Nominal data)
Cohort study
An observational study that recruits people with shared characteristics and follows them over time.
Confidence intervals (95%)
A range of values within which we are 95% confident that the true population value is situated.
Confirmability
A concept which refers to whether the data collected supports the conclusions drawn; used within qualitative studies.
Confounding factor/ variable
A variable that is linked to the dependent (outcome) variable and might influence the results obtained.
Control group
A group against which the effects of an intervention or the risk of developing a condition of interest are evaluated.

Cross-sectional study
An observational study characterised by collection of data at one point in time.
Experimental research (see Interventional research)
External validity (see Generalisability)
Focus group
Group discussions conducted in relation to a research focus.
Framework analysis
An approach to qualitative data analysis which utilises a thematic framework to organise and classify data according to key themes.
Generalisability
The extent to which findings from the research sample can be inferred to the wider population.
Intention-to-treat analysis
An approach to statistical analysis where participant's data is analysed according to the group they were allocated.
Internal validity
The extent to which a research study is thought to present the "truth" or the extent to which a research study is free of bias.
Interval data
Data that can be allocated to distinct ordered categories and the differences between categories is equal (compare Ordinal data).
Interventional research
Research where the research participants *are* exposed to treatment or intervention as part of the research (compare Observational research).
Longitudinal
A study characterised by collection of data over time (compare Cross-sectional).
Loss to follow-up
Failure to collect or absence of outcome data from research participants.
Meta-analysis
A quantitative combination of data.
Narrative synthesis
A qualitative, non-numerical, combination of data or themes from research studies.
Nominal data
Data that can be allocated to distinct categories but cannot be ordered (compare Ordinal data).
Non-randomised trial
An experimental study that does not allocate participants to groups using random methods (compare Randomised controlled trial).

Null hypothesis
The research statement you are looking to disprove, for example, there is no difference between treatments.

Observational research
Research where the participants *are not* exposed to treatment or intervention as part of the research (compare Interventional research).

Ordinal data
Data that can be allocated to ordered distinct categories, however the differences between categories are not equal (compare Nominal data).

P-value
Refers to the probability of obtaining the observed results if the null hypothesis is true.

Primary research
Research studies that collect data/ information directly from research participants.

Prospective
Looking forwards (compare Retrospective).

Publication bias
Systematic error attributable to publication status, for example non-publication of non-significant results.

Purposive sampling
Non-random method where participants are sampled according to a particular characteristic, for example experience of a service.

Qualitative research
Research that collects non-numerical data.

Qualitative synthesis (see Narrative synthesis)

Quantitative research
Research that collects numerical data.

Quasi-experimental study (see non-randomised trial)

Random allocation
A process where participants are assigned to groups using random (by chance) methods.

Randomised controlled trial
An experimental study where participants are allocated to intervention and control groups using random (by chance) methods to enable a comparative evaluation of treatment methods.

Ratio data
Data that can be allocated to distinct ordered categories and the differences between categories is equal with a true zero point being present (compare Interval data).

Recall bias
Systematic error attributable to a participants (in)ability to accurately recall past events.
Reflexivity
Refer to the role of the researcher in generating data.
Reliability
The extent to which different measures, tests, clinicians etc., agree.
Retrospective
Looking back (compare prospective).
Secondary research
Research studies, often called reviews, that collect data from primary studies.
Selection bias
Systematic error attributable to inadequate processes of recruitment and randomisation resulting in differences between groups at baseline.
Systematic review
Secondary research conducted using explicit methods including a transparent and comprehensive process of data retrieval, data collection, quality appraisal and data synthesis.
Thematic analysis
An approach to qualitative data analysis where themes are generated which reflect the data collected.
Triangulation
A process of comparison between different research methods and data to corroborate findings.
Uncontrolled trial
An experimental study that does not incorporate a control group.
Validity
The extent to which something represents what it is supposed to.

APPENDIX A

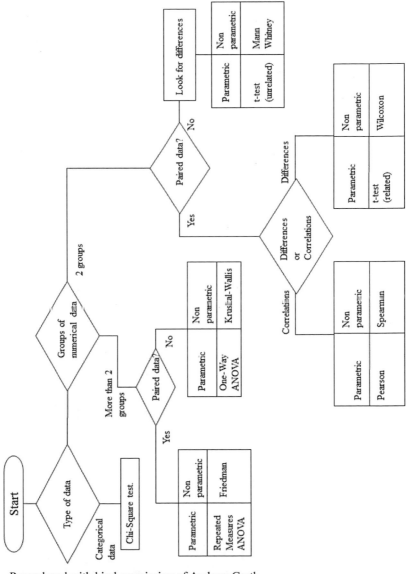

Reproduced with kind permission of Andrew Garth

INDEX